Career Chic

What Every Woman Should Know About Getting Ahead in Style

Carol Ann Pearce

illustrations by Elaine Yarbroudy

A PERIGEE BOOK
From Skylight Press

Perigee Books
are published by
The Putnam Publishing Group
200 Madison Avenue
New York, NY 10016

Copyright © 1990 by Skylight Press
Designed by Sheree L. Goodman

Library of Congress Cataloging-in-Publication Data

Pearce, Carol Ann.
    Career chic: what every woman should know about get-
ting ahead in style / by Carol Ann Pearce.
        p. cm.
    "A Perigee book."
    1. Clothing and dress. 2. Fashion. I. Title.
    ISBN 0-399-51576-3
    TT507.P36   1989   89-35279 CIP
    646'.34—dc20

Printed in the United States of America
1 2 3 4 5 6 7 8 9 10

Acknowledgments

I would like to thank the following people who generously offered their time, expertise, and creative good sense to this project:

Robin Brewster, advertising sales, *Life* magazine
Stella Flame, Stella Flame Boutique, New York
Phyllis Goodson, photographers' representative
Isa Irvin, hospital administrator
Misook Kim, Misook's Boutique, New York
Elizabeth Mauther, Hungarian Charities
Susan McCone, designer, Jonal Salon, New York
Maureen McTague, *The Washington Post*
Roseleen McTague, financial assistant, Memorial Sloan-Kettering Cancer Center, New York
Sandi Mendelson, president, Hilsinger/Mendelson, Inc.
Charlotte Moore, chancellor, International Academy of Merchandising and Design
Deborah Rose O'Neal, teacher
Victoria Pik, merchandising executive, London Fog
Bonnie Reichman, M.D.
Mary Ann Seduski, advertising manager, AT&T
Julie Siegel, recruiter, Chase Manhattan Bank
Connie Skidmore, tax partner, Coopers & Lybrand, Los Angeles
Wendi Winters, The Rowland Company, New York
Barbara Wood, psychiatric social worker, New York

Special thanks to my husband for his unflagging encouragement and support.

Contents

Career Chic

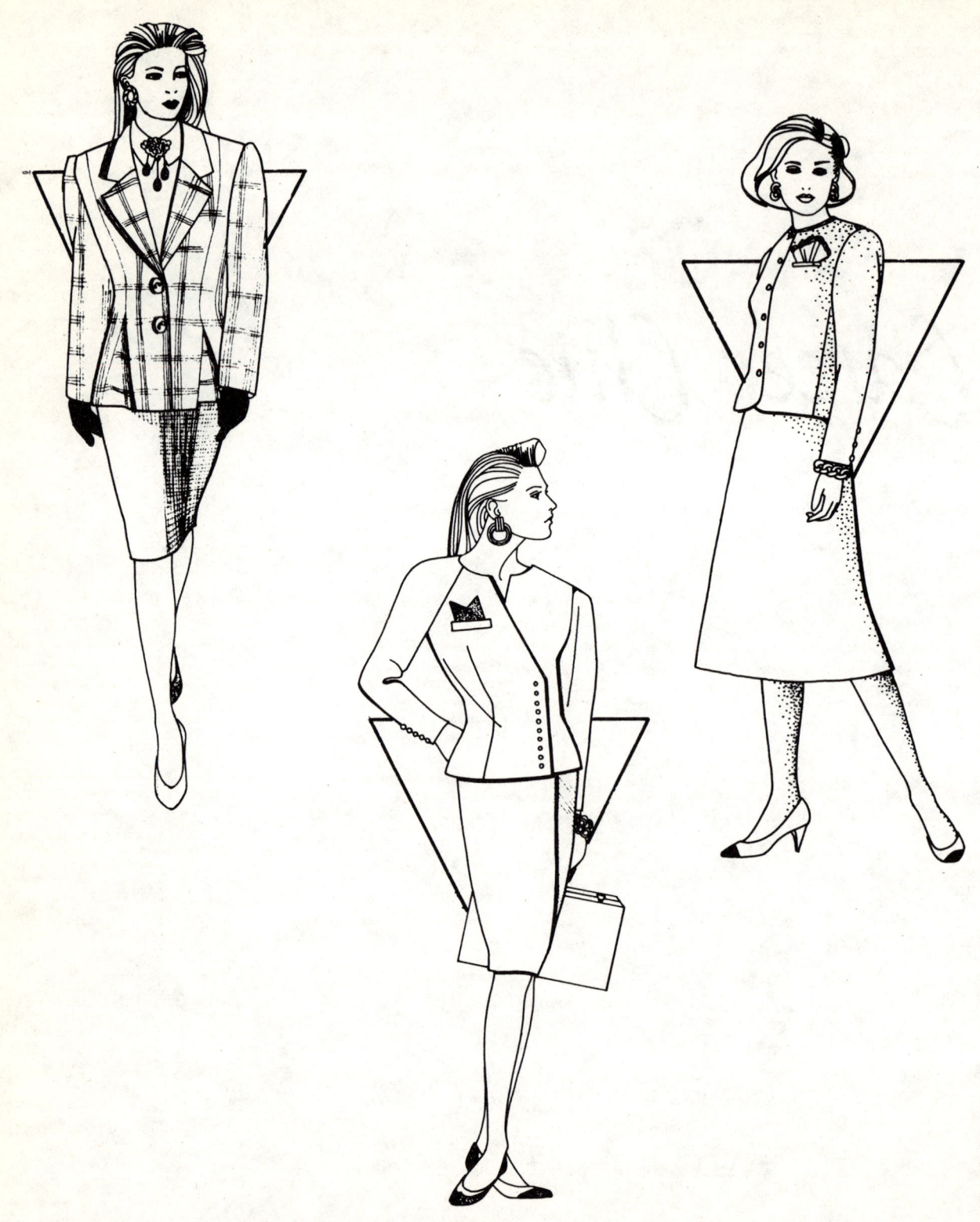

The New Power Dressing

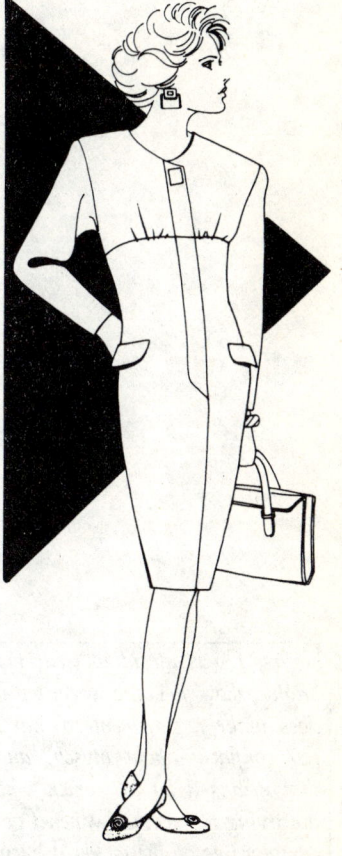

Professional women have worked hard and long to get where they are today. Take a look around. We've chalked up a multitude of solid successes and carved out an entirely new place for ourselves in the job market. Women are now taken seriously in almost all fields, including formerly exclusive-male bastions such as international finance, law, and accounting. In a whole range of businesses throughout the workplace, we are at last reaping some real rewards. Nevertheless, this is no time to relax. What brought us success yesterday, may not keep us there tomorrow. Everything we do, every move we make, every thought we think must be as up-to-date as possible. In short, it is time to reassess one of the tools we used to get us this far. And that is FASHION.

What did it actually do for us? It helped us appear professional to those who might, merely because of our gender, have concluded otherwise. And how did it do this? To put it bluntly, fashion either helped us look like men, or at the very least helped us reflect what men felt women should look like in the workplace—as if our competence and talents could not speak loudly enough on their own.

But times have changed. We've proved ourselves, and most of our male employees, counterparts, and bosses now enjoy and respect our business personas.

We have entered a new era, and once again, fashion stands

Says one lawyer: "There has to be a certain nod toward convention, and if you're going to be dealing with clients who tend to be older men, you'll probably have to dress conservatively; but there are a lot of choices in the range between a red silk dress and what's appropriate. It may take a woman a long time to come to this, where she can say, 'I can be my own kind of person,' but it's worth it in the long run."

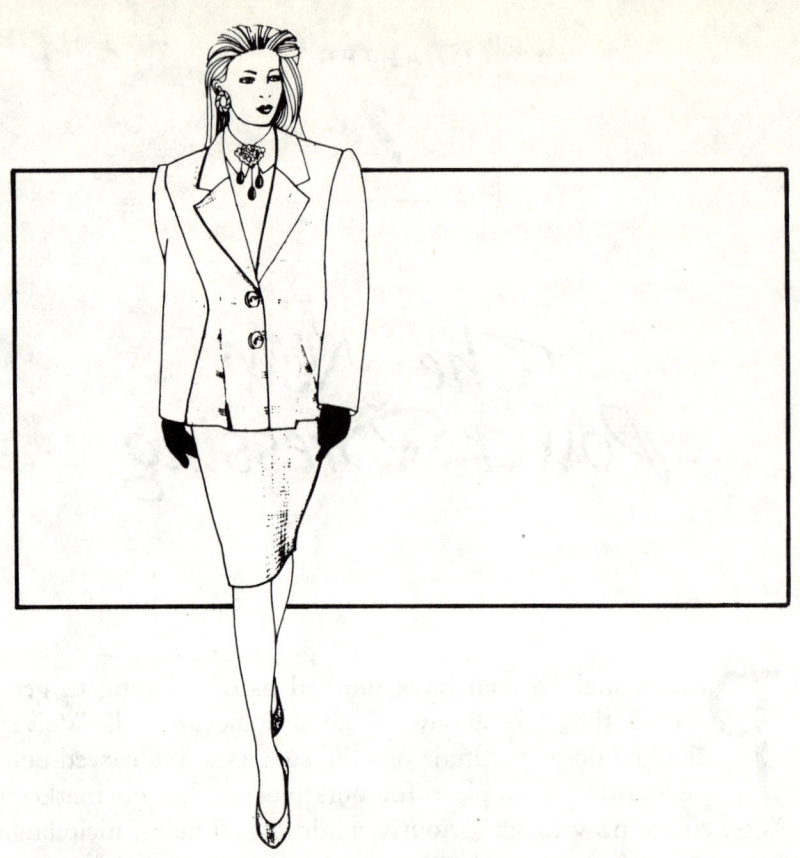

before us as a tool. It can help us truly present ourselves with all the uniqueness, strength, and color we bring to our work. And best of all, we can allow it to express our professional yet *feminine* selves.

The éclat we've achieved has now brought a cornucopia of fashion options. When starting out, unproven, you're constrained by rules, but when you're strong and capable and people know it, you have more freedom to choose.

At this stage, women are no longer required to look a certain way to overcome resistance in the workplace. No longer do we have to hide the fact that we are a) feminine and b) individual by hiding behind a stiff suit. We can be taken as serious business women while looking exquisitely female. We can even go so far as to look correctly and appropriately "alluring" (but not "sexy") without detracting from a competent, professional image. That's how far we've come, and that's a long, long way.

Now it's up to each of us individually to take advantage of this chance to dress and look female, to set aside the corseting constrictions of yesterday's dress-for-success rules, to seize the new-won freedoms, and to dress in a way that is professionally feminine and attractive, and uniquely and smashingly ourselves.

If this sounds chancy, consider this: Some firms today actually require women executives to break the old dress codes and are issuing reminders that urge women to "look great every day." From hospitals in the midwest to finance institutions in the far west to fashion and beauty boutiques in the south, women are being encouraged to invest in attractive, feminine clothes. One firm has gone so far as to give each woman employee $100 cash and a $250 interest-free loan toward a new wardrobe. The change is upon us. The freedom—and the time to look spectacular—is here. Career dressing no longer automatically means menswear. The uniform of yesterday is history and clinging to it will simply mean that the promotion parade could pass you by.

These are the new principles: Boring is out. Prim is out. Dull is out. Mannish is out. Severe—out. The safe gray suit with the pale-blue blouse and speck earrings—out. The pin-striped suit with the narrow tie and librarian shoes—out. Color is here. Accessories are everywhere. Movement in fabric and styling is downright de rigueur. For some of us, it may take a while to accept the fact and to take the chance on wearing previously forbidden styles and colors. With prestige and salary on the line, it's always hard to let go of what worked in the past.

So to prove to yourself that the fashion water is safe, look around. What do you see? No more gray mice, no more corporateers. Granted, with patience and telescopic vision you might pick out a few pockets of yesterday's dressers, but not many, and not for long. Mostly those still playing it "safe" are the entry-level brigade, desperately playing by rules they think they can't afford to ignore.

For the most part, you will see that women just like you are expanding their dress codes according to what they want. They are deciding for themselves what is appropriate within certain career boundaries, ignoring past notions which are alien to them.

Of course different businesses allow for different possibilities.

From the accounting profession, a VP reports that annual evaluation reviews will soon include a rejoinder that women begin to show some creativity and personal style in their business dress. "Men are sick of seeing younger women in bow ties and white shirts," she said, not mentioning the fact that most women are sick of seeing themselves in these uniforms as well.

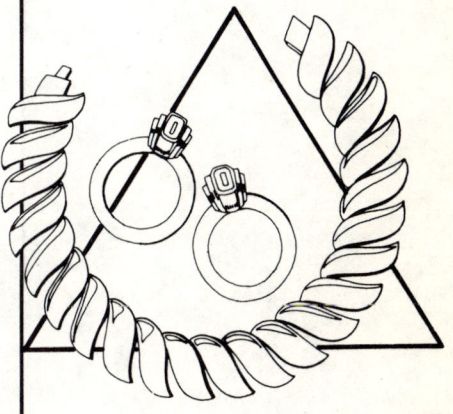

Within each field, you will find certain fashion parameters, and what works beautifully for, say a design consultant, would be disaster for a loan officer in an investment firm. In some career fields, women are wearing red dresses to board meetings. In banking this would be the equivalent of showing up in pajamas. With new power dressing, it is important to pay close attention to the atmosphere created by your own field and to dress within those limits. Within those boundaries, however, there is plenty of room to be who you are as a woman and as an individual.

The only limit is one's own imagination, and, given the extent of women's accomplishments to date, our imaginations have already proven to be one of the best friends we have.

Don't hold back. Nothing can make a woman look as out of date, as unsophisticated, as professionally over-the-hill as yesterday's fashion uniform. This book will guide you in making choices, will help you test yourself out in the newness of this changing career chic. The chapters that follow hold a wealth of tips to show you step by step how to know the difference between what's appropriate and what is too overdone or too understated to be effective. There are also pointers on ways to update what you already have in your closet even *if* it's a gray mouse suit. By the end of this book, you'll be trusting your own instincts in shopping and coordinating a look, even when it comes to the hard-to-work-with separates for mismatched styles that combine such things as stripes and polka dots!

Few of us were born with an innate ability to choose the clothes that are right for us or just the right accessories with the right garments. This is a skill that comes with thought, practice, and a little help from these pages. It's not difficult and it is immensely rewarding. Once you've mastered the premises in this book, you will be able to look professionally chic and stunningly feminine under any and all challenging business circumstances from the company picnic to a presentation in L.A.

The New Picture

There are so many fashion options now that we don't have to cling to that short list of permissible items like the gray suit, black pumps, and white handkerchief. Forget that outmoded list. Use the following hints in order to get familiar with your own particular professional needs, restrictions, and preferences. What's right for somebody else may not be right for you. That's part of the new power dressing: Your way is the only right way for you, and only you can make those decisions. The key is to make them with confidence and intelligence. Toward that goal keep this key principle in mind:

> It's not the extent of your wardrobe that counts. It's what it looks like that matters. To this end, always buy the very best you can afford. Choose at least a few classic lines and neutral colors in basic garments such as suits, jackets, and skirts. This quality fashion bedrock will guarantee that when you're putting together a look, you will always look terrific.

Designer Cathy Hardwick recommends working with just ten to twelve pieces in an entire wardrobe, pieces that will work in any situation. That includes several jackets, three to four skirts, the same number of blouses, and perhaps a dress or two. Looking distinguished with this kind of an approach is not just feasible, it's just about surefire. Then with just a few special touches, you move from merely looking distinguished to looking absolutely fantastic.

Putting It All Together

Let's dive right into the key general guidelines that will start you in the right fashion direction. Throughout the book we will illustrate in words and pictures the points below. But for now, read them over, and allow these observations to begin the job of expanding your fashion vision.

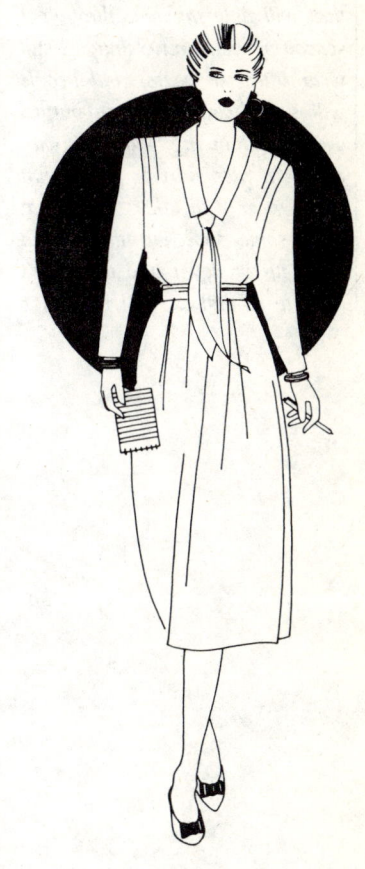

TV star Amanda Pays feminizes her look primarily with belts and confident thrift-shop forays for just the right accessories. She describes her L.A. look as "eclectic."

- Clothes conveying movement, fullness, curved lines, fitted waists, softness, and femininity are in.

- What you feel best in is what you build on, be it fabric, cut, or color—or all three, so long as you keep your eye on the best possible quality you can afford.

- Jackets can now show off, rather than conceal, figure lines such as waists. Take special care in choosing a jacket and go for quality fabric and at least one or two with classic lines. This still gives you free rein to go with collarless, collared, double-breasted, single-breasted, off-center closing, single button—in short, a wide range of simple yet classic possibilities. The jacket is the most important part of any business wardrobe. Make sure it fits perfectly. Have it tailored if necessary. You can change fashion looks completely with a good jacket; dress it up or down with jewelry and other accessories. Buy a jacket that will last for many seasons.

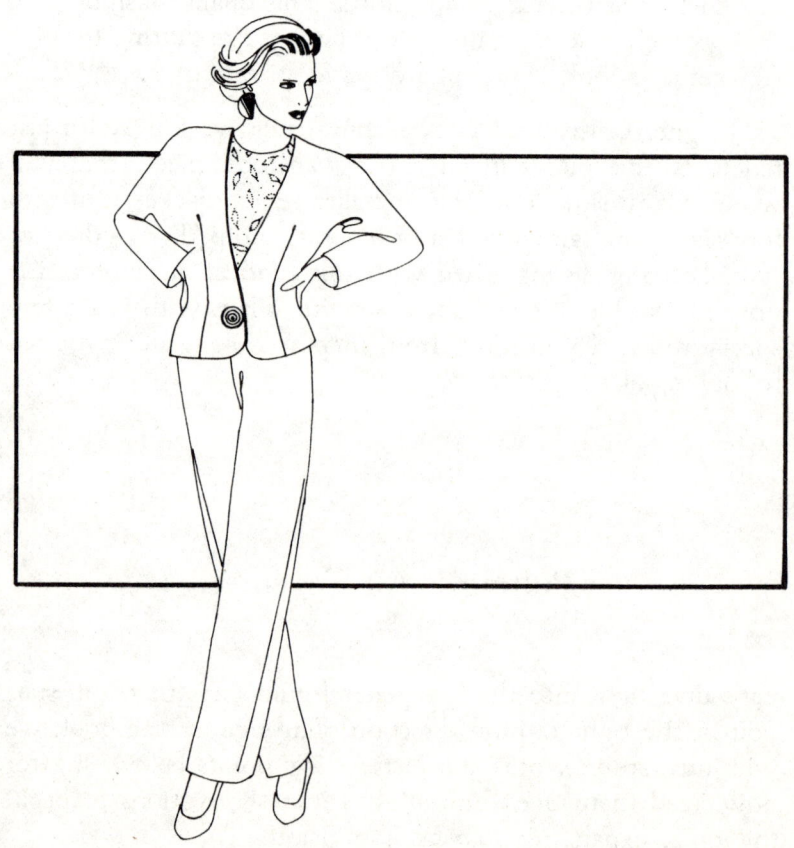

- Skirts have come a long way from the pencil line, and that's just fine for business. The whole range of choices from pleats and tiers of pleats to wraps work well.

- Hemlines are up, they're in between, they're down, depending on personal preference and attributes. The important principle is: Avoid extremes. Some short hemlines (upper to mid-knee) are showing up without a repercussion in certain fields. In other professions, skirts to the bottom of the knee are about as short as one can go. If you don't know how short is too short, just look at what executive women in your business are wearing.

    Dresses move strongly into this new picture of career chic. They now come with jackets which gives a unique suited look. Or they come with a flower pin which promotes a feminine look. Very soon, dresses should be coming in an even greater variety of fabrics and styles as designers respond to women's needs and demands.

- Separates gear up to the stylishly iconoclastic "un-matched suit" look which requires mixing and matching. Developing an eye for what items work together, including such things as pindots and stripes, is a talent to be cultivated. Once mastered, however, mixing and matching can turn a few clothes into a wide variety of choices which is why so many women prefer separates.

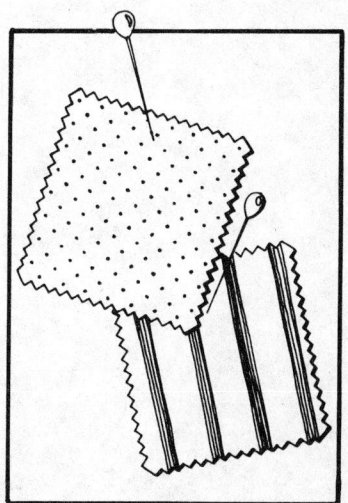

- Pants are back. They are soft and full and add another fashion choice to the work wardrobe. Many businesses do frown on women wearing pants, yet women are slowly, cautiously returning to pants suits for work, while avoiding anything that conveys a masculine image. If pants are worn, they should be part of an elegant suit, with some glamorous accessories.

- Blouses can keep up the power pace with details such as cream-on-cream embroidery, full romantic sleeves, brilliant colors, and they're available today in easy-care yet silky fabrics. They don't have to be silk to have the best possible effect, but silk is still the staple of the new power dressing.

- Accessories add a different character to any business outfit and can change a daytime look into a nighttime dinner meeting. They must be bold enough to be noticed. Don't go for background effect. The scale in accessories can definitely be larger than in the past. Large gold earrings are appearing on the business scene, along with long, loopy beads, clunky necklaces, and antique brooches.

- Scarves should be expensive ones that will last and that reflect a quality look, expertly wrapped, tied, or draped.

- Shoes—and even boots—come with bows, as well as in vivid colors and patterns. The power pump is still a classy choice, and plain hose are also beautifully classic. Still, you will find that the classic pump exhibits the right amount of flair if it carries a geometric slash of color or some other idiosyncratic detail that conveys both quality and originality.

- All one-color outfits don't work as well as an experimentation with shades and combinations. Brilliant splashes of such unlikely hues as chartreuse and fuchsia punctuate a look, give it that all-important up-to-date "together" impact. Learn which colors enhance your complexion in order to keep from looking exhausted on overtime days.

Keep in mind that there is no rigid right or wrong way to dress for success anymore. Establishing what's right for your

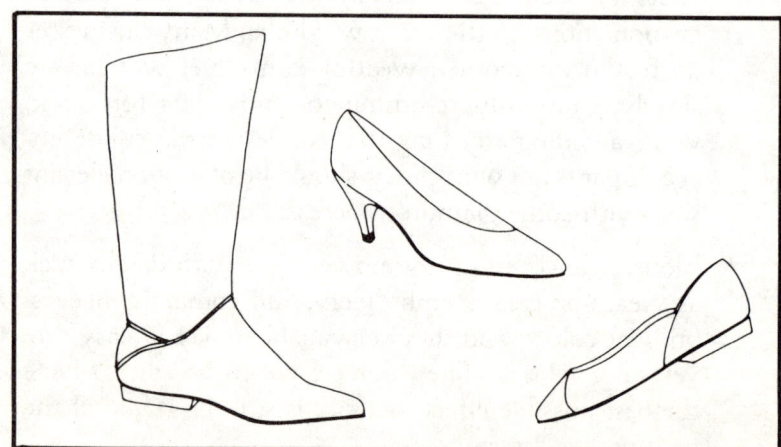

professional image and then making it *personal* are the new power-dressing goals. And when you feel good about how you look, you will wear the look with grace and verve.

Know Yourself

For those used to "uniform" dressing, the adjustment may not come easily. Of course, going with current fashions is not the answer because that's simply exchanging one set of constrictions for another. Everyone needs to find what works for them.

Ask yourself these key questions. The answers will help guide you toward your own special needs and style.

1. What is your professional style? Just because other women look like they stepped out of "L.A. Law" doesn't mean this is the right style for you. You might be the more feminine Jane Pauley business type. Try and remember an outfit that made you feel particularly confident. Break it down into its parts.

2. What cuts look good on you? What lines hide those aspects of your body you consider figure flaws?

3. What can you afford? Remember, skimping on basics is a big mistake. Far better to have less options in your closet than many wrong ones. Shopping discount designer houses is a smart move.

4. When buying garments, do your choices have built-in longevity? They should. Current fashions that may be out of style next year represent a poor investment. Few of us who work can afford to change our wardrobe every few years. Let classic basics be the foundation which you update and enhance through accessories.

5. What do you have in your closets now? Hold on to those classic suits and blazers, to silk blouses and skirts in neutral colors, with good cuts or made from exquisite fabrics. Give away everything else. Paring down allows you to see what you really have to work with. A clutter of

A hospital administrator states: "Even in the most conservative fields where you really are genuinely constrained, I believe there is still room to turn yourself out as other than a cookie-cutter replica of your male colleague."

leftovers only clouds those early morning decisions about what to wear and what to put with another item.

Striking the
Feminine/Business Balance

Even though we are enjoying a new freedom, there are still some good fashion rules that will probably always be with us. Here's a quick look at that fine and all-important line between appropriate and inappropriate, the details of which will be explored throughout this book. Smart wear is (and probably always will be):

- Expensive enough to convey quality but not so overdone as to announce, "I've got money."

- Formal but not so stiff as to appear severe and intimidating.

- Chic but not so trendy as to convey a lack of steadiness.

- Feminine but not so feminine as to reflect more of an interest in "prettiness" than "business."

- Mature but not matronly so as to convey a conservativeness mixed with fresh ideas.

- Up-to-date but not so youthful or schoolgirlish as to appear cute not competent.

- Comfortable without being casual, which does not convey high stakes.

- A bold statement but not loud. Mice don't win. Neither do gaudy eyefuls.

New Priorities

Let's prioritize the new mind-set. What does this all add up to for today's career woman on-the-go and on-the-rise? Pared down to basics, this is what counts:

New Priorities for the New Power Dressing

- Appropriateness
- Individuality
- An expanding definition of the executive look
- A strong statement
- Softness, femininity
- Bold colors both as accents and key items
- A lean wardrobe with every item packing a punch
- Unique accessories that draw attention
- Proportion
- Quality
- Timelessness

The "L.A. Law" look is one of conservative yet feminine suits with classy silk blouses.

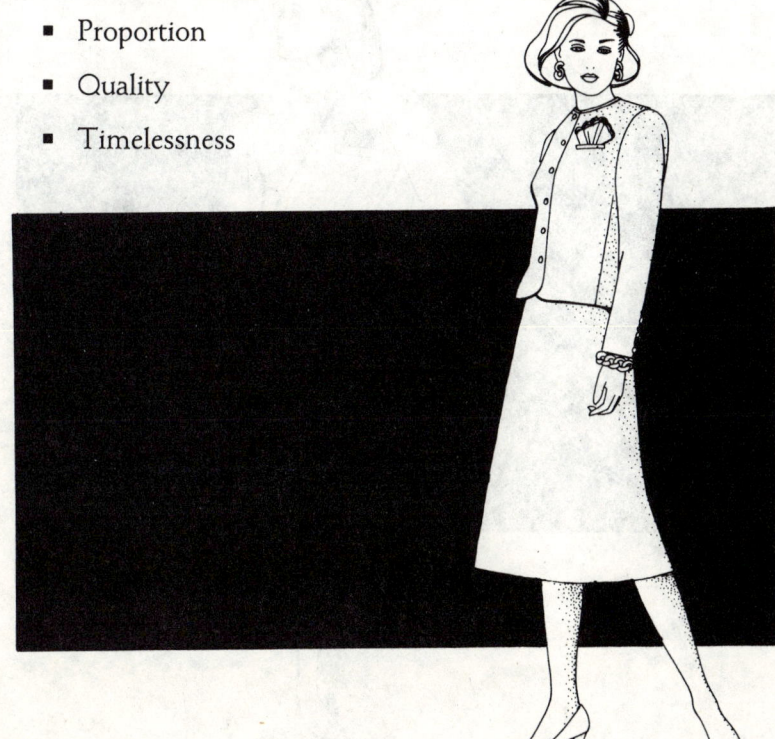

Creating the professional image through the way we carry ourselves and the way we dress is anything but a frivolous matter. In the business world, appearance is a good part of the battle. We are perceived to be doing a good job if we *look* as though we're competent and capable. If our dress is sloppy, outmoded, mousy, we will be judged in that light. From the crucial job interview all the way on up the success ladder, how we look, how we dress, will be one of the prime ways in which we convey the impression of our talents.

Looking superb will also have a salutary effect on our own psyches at the same time. If we're wearing a black-on-black woven rayon designer skirt with a carefully "mismatched" imported woven rayon black on ice-white collarless jacket with exquisitely detailed pockets and rows of tiny black pearl but-

"I think you should dress every day as if you were going to speak to the president of the company."
Administrator

"I feel that how you feel about yourself is related to how you perform, so women who undercut themselves, underplay how they look, and don't feel good about their appearance, I don't think they can do their best work."
Investment Banker

tons at the cuffs, clunky gold earrings, and a pair of black and white spectator "power" pumps, a lacy handkerchief barely peeping out of a breast pocket, who is going to convince us that we don't know what we're talking about?

In short, if we *look* the part, people, including ourselves, will believe we can *play* the part. It may sound simplistic, but even in business, when we look sharp, whatever we do is going to be perceived as savvy. Dressing smart sends out a clear message to those who control career promotions: We know what we're doing and nobody can do it better.

This book tells you all you need to know in order to achieve the new power dressing. Try our tips on achieving your own polished and particular look, and follow important Dos and Don'ts until you find your own footing. You will be amazed at the effectiveness of a fashion look that sings your praises.

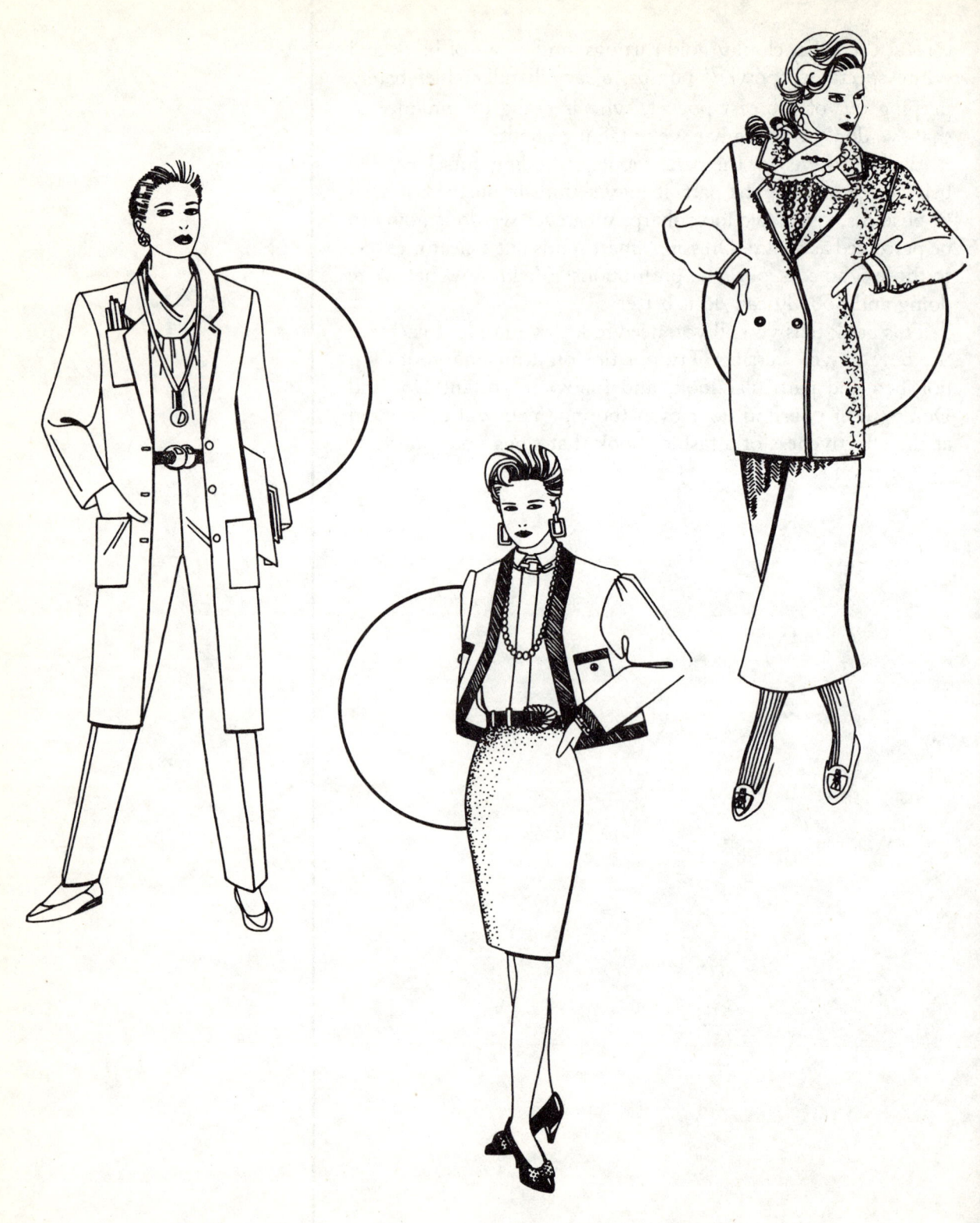

Playing the Field

While fashion standards change in the business world, and while a personal, idiosyncratic statement is one of the most contemporary assertions you can make, how far to go with this freedom depends on the field in which you carve out your career. The gamut ranges from ultraconservative to trendy, although even the very ultra are not so conservative now as they used to be.

Says one executive, "Professions break down by how creative they are. The more creative, the less conservative and the more freedom there is to indulge your own personality."

Wall Street, law, finance, and banking tip the conservative scale, although bear in mind that even they are not so pinstriped as in years past. Publishing, fashion merchandising, the creative areas of advertising, teaching, and social work appear at the opposite pole with more flexibility and even some allowance for a touch of the trendy. Spread along the middle area are such fields as advertising management, public relations, and, believe it or not, accounting.

What influences fashion choices within each of these separate fiefdoms are such factors as the clients you handle, the people you report to (and their tastes), the degree of spotlight you receive within and without the company, the work you do, and the area of the field within which you work.

For example, advertising in itself accommodates a reach of

Katie Kelly, NBC movie critic, highlights her full white/gray hair with white-and-black patterned jackets.

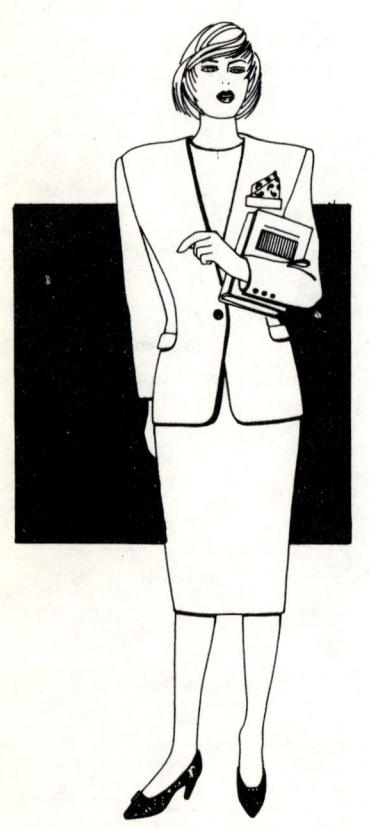

*P*hylicia Rashad as Claire Huxtable in "The Cosby Show" wore a bright-yellow, long-line, double-breasted jacket with a pencil-slim skirt on a sequence that showed her at her law office.

dress codes. Account executives who deal directly with clients dress as prudently as any Wall Streeter. Within the same firm, the creative director may show up for work in a white shirt and jeans. Another executive in the firm with young, trendy clients to please will probably wear mismatched separates, bright colors, and if it suits her, shorter hemlines.

The reason behind these differences lies in the way the various professions are perceived. Accountants are expected to convey a stolid prudence, a convervatism that one hopes extends to the way they handle cash. Lawyers, similarly, strive to convey a solidarity, a rock of jurisprudence quality, which, in turn, reassures clients as to their ability to move legal megamountains. Both these fields convey that facts, not creativity, are their business. Art directors, on the other hand, and depending on the context, want to communicate just the opposite. They should reflect creativity. Often the more offbeat and eccentric the attire, without going completely overboard, the better. Such looks say, "I'm filled with ideas." At a corporate meeting, however, this same art director might wear an impressively classic suit (with just a subtle hint of eccentricity in a well-chosen accessory) that would proclaim, "I'm inventive, but I also know the game and can play it with the best of them."

Here's what some successful people in their fields are doing.

Law

- "This is not quite the 'L.A. Law' scene, as neophytes tend to stick to the gray or navy flannel, man-tailored suits which they feel they must wear in order to be suitably dressed. Which isn't true at all," says a lawyer who has been in the field for a number of years. "The young lawyers who dress that way don't feel good about themselves. They admit the look isn't flattering or attractive, but they think it's what they have to do. That's curious, because you're talking about women with bright minds, you would think they could apply that perceptiveness to the way they look, but they're afraid to take the chance. Where they work is still conservative and old-world."

- "Generally women in law dress conservatively, but I have seen some wearing unmatched suits, for example. I don't think lawyers can or should wear pants, but short of that, I don't believe we're restricted as to color. I've worn a red blouse with a black skirt. A lot of women think they can't wear this type of clothing out of fear that they won't be distinguished from the secretaries, but I say if they spend three hundred and seventy-five dollars for a flannel skirt and four hundred dollars for a sweater, nobody will be confused as to who's who."

Accounting—West Coast

- "In accounting, we're not hemmed in by narrow choices anymore. Mostly I wear suits which is what the women around me wear also, but not the traditional suit of five years ago. That is, not the dark pin-striped suit with a bow tie. The accounting blue-and-white uniform is definitely out. I've been with my firm for eleven years now and have made partner, and I wear a lot of unmatched suits. I even have a bright-red suit. I hesitated to wear it, but it worked out very well."

- "I wear a lot of scarves and jewelry. I feel I'm having an influence in my office, which is the San Francisco Bay area. More women are dressing this way around me now, getting away from the boring clothes we've all been wearing to work."

- "We had our annual evaluation several weeks ago, and men were telling me that they would like women to stop thinking they have to be just like a man in order to succeed. However, I don't wear pants or dresses to work. I prefer suits and separates."

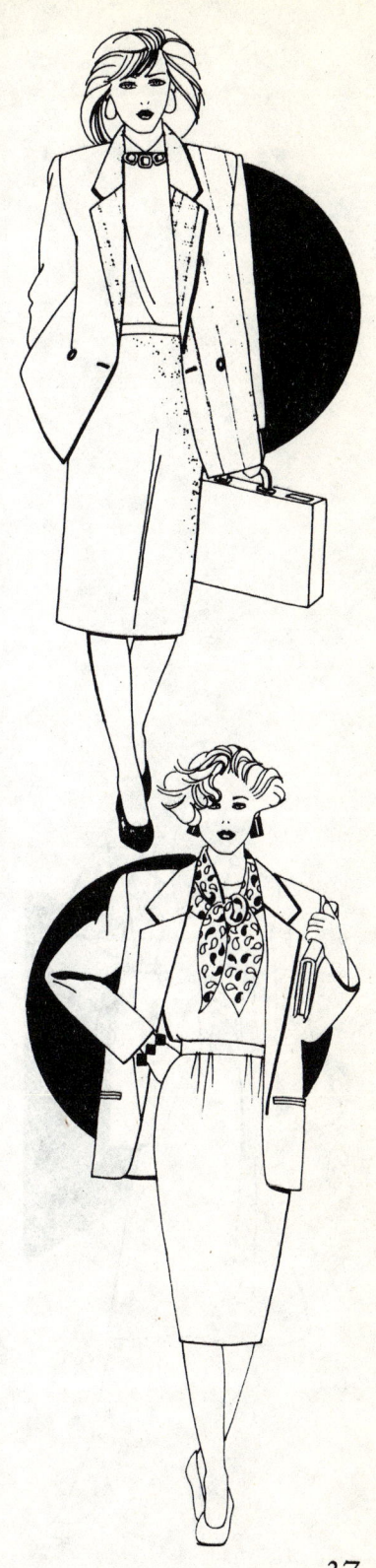

Banking

- "Sometimes I wear a red suit which has an oversize jacket with huge buttons, and that's okay. I wear a white shirt with it which tones it down, makes it more acceptable, and pearl earrings. I don't want to go too far; you can't be too flashy in banking. At the same time, if you're high-up enough, you have a lot more leeway. One of our VPs wore a lavender linen suit the other day and she looked great."

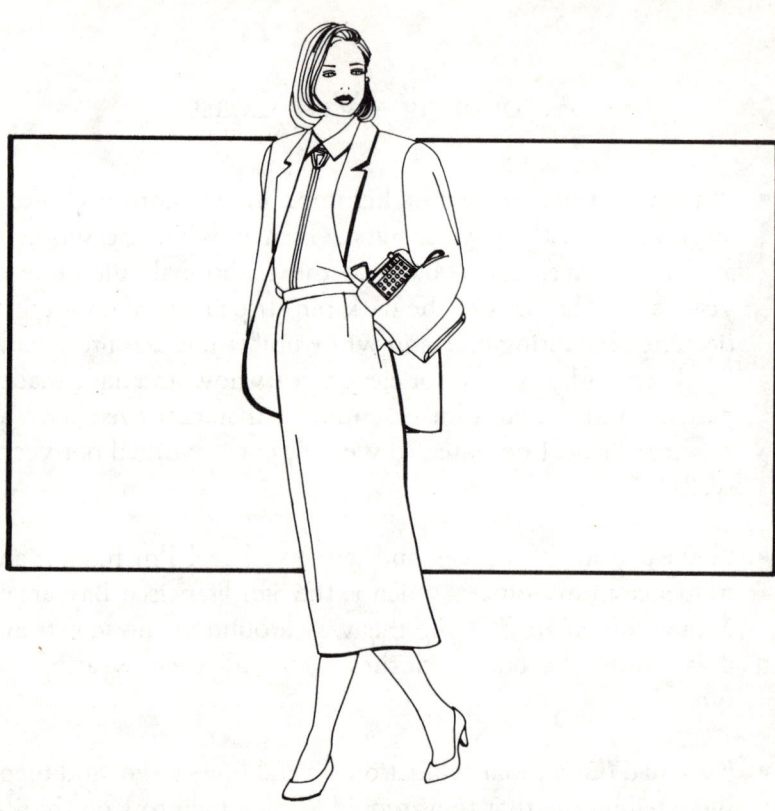

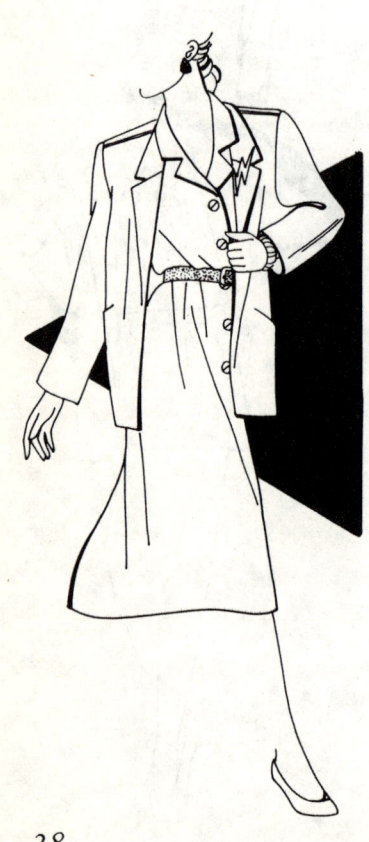

- "We used to subscribe to the gray mice syndrome in banking, but no more. There's also no need to look masculine anymore, and I don't see women doing that. For interviews, though, you have to dress very conservatively, which is probably true in most fields. When I interviewed for this job, they called me in at the last minute and I said, "I'm wearing a red blouse." So they checked to see if that would be okay, and it was all right, but what that did show was that I was aware of the rules. But once you get that job, you look around and see what others in the department wear. That's how you gauge yourself then."

- "Even in banking, though, we like people to show some individuality. Suits with some coloring work, not just gray or black which shows so little imagination. And maybe some style in accessories—not so much pearls anymore but bigger jewelry. Again, you can't wear these to an interview but in the workplace. Subdued colors work best for an interview."

- "Maybe once a week I wear a dress to work, and I keep a jacket at the office in case I have to see the VP on something. And I always wear stockings, even in summer, even if I'm tanned. In summer I also tend to wear linen suits though they do wrinkle. Somebody just came to my door looking very wrinkled, but linen is supposed to wrinkle so we walk around looking like we slept in our clothes, but that's fine because linen is a classic fabric and supposed to look that way. This wouldn't have been acceptable five years ago, but now it's okay because linen is a quality fabric and not stiff. Actually rayon is easier on wrinkling—in general, the blends are better."

- "I see myself going to bigger buttons, skirts to my knee, bigger jackets, and more dresses. I would not wear knit dresses, and would wear sweaters only if they looked like a blouse—and then not very often."

Corporate Management

- "I believe it pays to buy expensive garments as the quality of clothing is important. Clothes should be out of good fabrics or well styled so they can be worn different ways, rather than buying inexpensive items that don't fit properly or wear well and never do look that good even from the beginning."

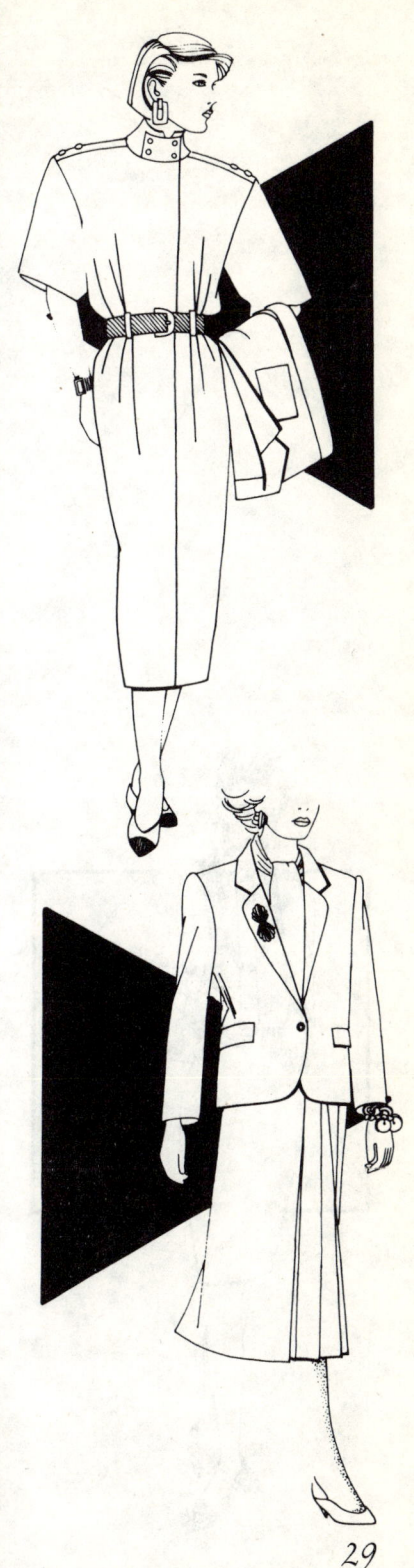

29

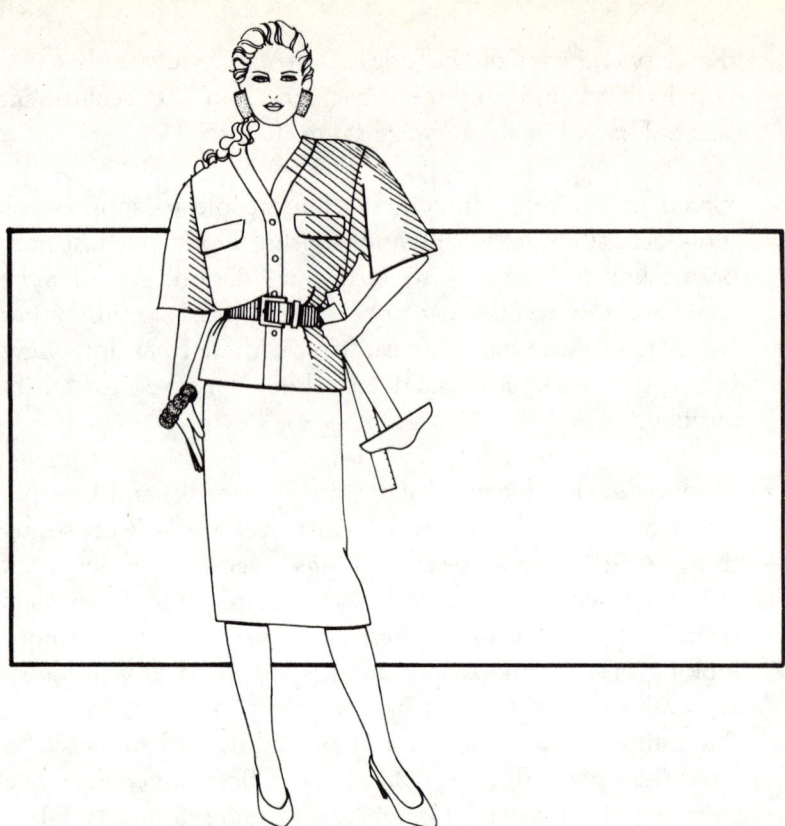

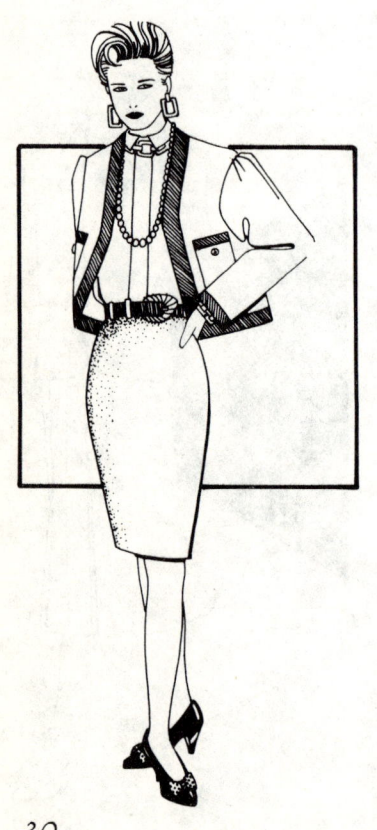

- "Usually I wear a suit or dress with a jacket in a different color—no gray or navy anymore. I might wear a yellow or bright-red jacket with a black or gray skirt. Or I'll wear a burgundy blouse with a yellow jacket. Earrings are important, too, because people really notice them. Gold earrings, a gold necklace and bracelet pull things together beautifully."

- "In winter I wear V-neck silk blouses like those worn in 'L.A. Law.' I like that look. In summer, I wear a silk short-sleeved or linen blouse, silk because I like the dressy way it feels and because it doesn't go out of style and looks feminine."

- "Our sales people generally wear a kind of 'uniform' consisting of a navy suit and white or light-blue shirt and tie. The emphasis there is to appear as a conservative businessperson to the customer. Women still follow in men's footsteps in the sales force, and flamboyance is not the image there. I don't see women wearing pants in business, though.

I don't think they're acceptable. As for hemlines, I do see skirts about the knee but no real minis. For myself, I wear no deep necklines and always wear a jacket. My overall guidelines are clothes that are flattering and make me feel attractive."

Advertising

- "I see everything from jeans to slacks with sweaters and suits with open-collared blouses—all quality, not just the very expensive—in advertising agencies when I make rounds with a portfolio. As for myself, I generally wear something like a belted silk overblouse with a really good, slim-line skirt, or in summer, I might wear a white linen skirt with a black raw-silk overblouse that looks like a light jacket. I prefer mixing and matching because it's versatile."

- "I basically buy in beige, ivory, and black—classic colors. That makes it easier to mix and match. For example, I just bought a black designer suit in lightweight wool, and I'll be able to wear the jacket from it with plaid skirts, with slacks, and with other colors, too."

- "I do a lot of walking so I wear medium heels. When it rains, I just wear my shoes anyway and don't worry about them. Or I wear a pair of short black suede boots that get wet but still look good. My trench coat is water resistant and I carry a wonderful big umbrella."

- "I've been wearing more dresses lately, but still most of my business wear consists of suits. I soften them with silk blouses—no bow ties—pearl earrings, shoes with possibly slingback heels. I wear higher heels now, too. I used to wear sneakers walking to work but no more. I don't like that look."

- "At one time I was the real 'corporateer'—wearing conservative tailored business suits with bow ties. Look in the

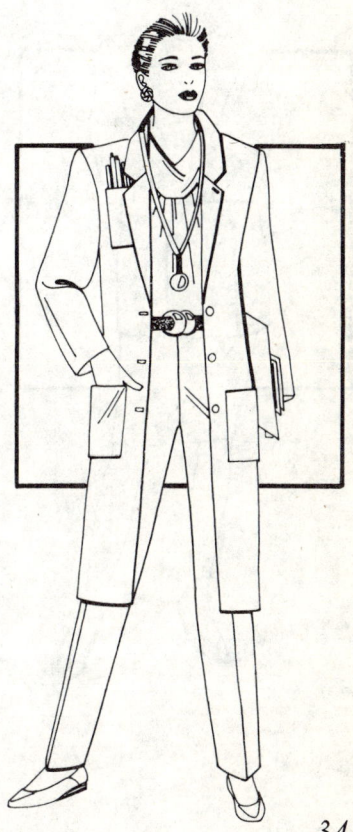

Connie Chung, of CBS News, favors dresses, sometimes with wide, bold collars and at other times, a little-girl look with huge white collars, short sleeves, and white cuffs. Occasionally, however, she also sports a turtleneck with a collarless suit.

31

mirror, I would see a corporateer looking back at me. Now I go for softer looks because you can be professional and still be feminine. I've started to give away my straight suits because it's much more fun mixing and matching. Within boundaries, I find there is a lot you can do that is your own. Occasionally I wear pants, but not often."

- "Today I'm wearing a black linen skirt with a crisp white blouse, a white blazer, a wide black designer belt with a gold buckle, pearl earrings, a long pearl necklace and a gold choker, pale-white hose, medium-heeled pumps with a polka-dot bow on the toe and a white stripe on the heel. They're Italian and very comfortable."

Medical

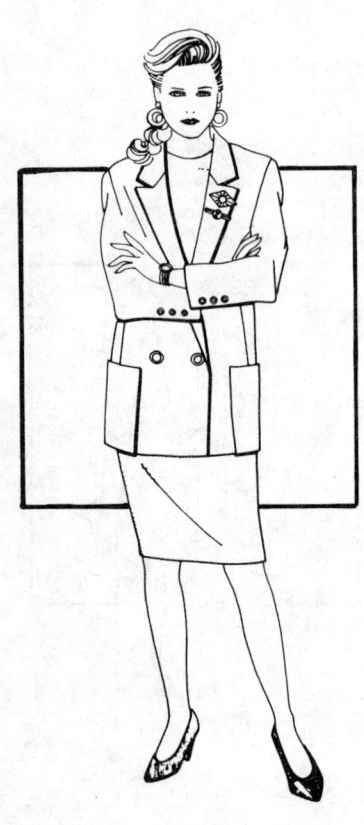

- "I wear a whole range of things so long as I feel comfortable and look as good as I can. You have to remember that doctors in a hospital setting are always wearing these white coats, so whatever I put on is geared to having the white coat over it. I wear suits but I usually slip off the jacket before I slip on the white coat. Often I even wear pants. My shoes have to have medium-to-low heels because I'm on my feet a lot making rounds or in the hospital clinic."

- "I have some houndstooth plaid and glen plaid slacks that I wear with silk blouses and a wide belt which I like very much."

- "Mostly I wear dresses, once in a while a suit. I know that patients like you to look official, so I would never wear anything casual. My shoes have medium heels, my dress sleeves are always long, even in summertime. I would not wear a skirt shorter than the bottom of my knee either. I think this is fine perhaps for women in less serious professions, but when you deal with people's health, they have to regard you as someone of weight—not frivolous. I see some doctors in hospitals, especially if they are young, wear

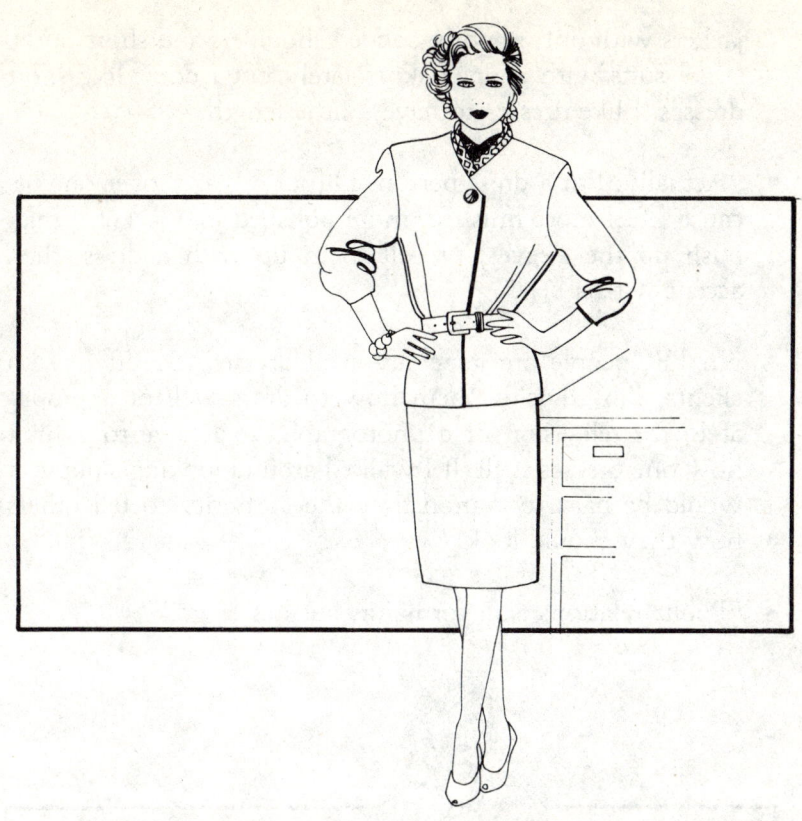

short skirts. Perhaps in that setting it is all right, but I'm not sure. Having my own practice, I set my own standards and I stick to a more mature and serious impression in my dress."

Public Relations

- "I feel most comfortable dressed in my version of what's appropriate, and that means basically suits and dresses that are somewhat formal but unstructured. I collect antique clips which I may clip onto a neckline or a suit lapel. The clips are from the '40s, and I may wear pairs of them or just one. I think they add a unique touch."

- "In suits, I choose classic lines, no style extremes such as the peplum suit popular now, although I am wearing longer jackets with only slightly padded shoulders and short skirts. I like suits with shorter skirts lately but I don't like short dresses. I like dresses to have a little length."

- "Actually, I'm a dress person. I'll put a blazer over one because I feel more finished, more polished in a jacket. I may push up the sleeves, or roll them up with a dress, then accent with a belt."

- "In PR, people are generally well dressed. So often with clients, I'm advising them how to dress well or appropriately for television or a photograph, so I have to exhibit how one dresses well. If I walked around looking sloppy, it would be hard to demonstrate the authority to tell others how they should look."

- "Public relations isn't formal as businesses go."

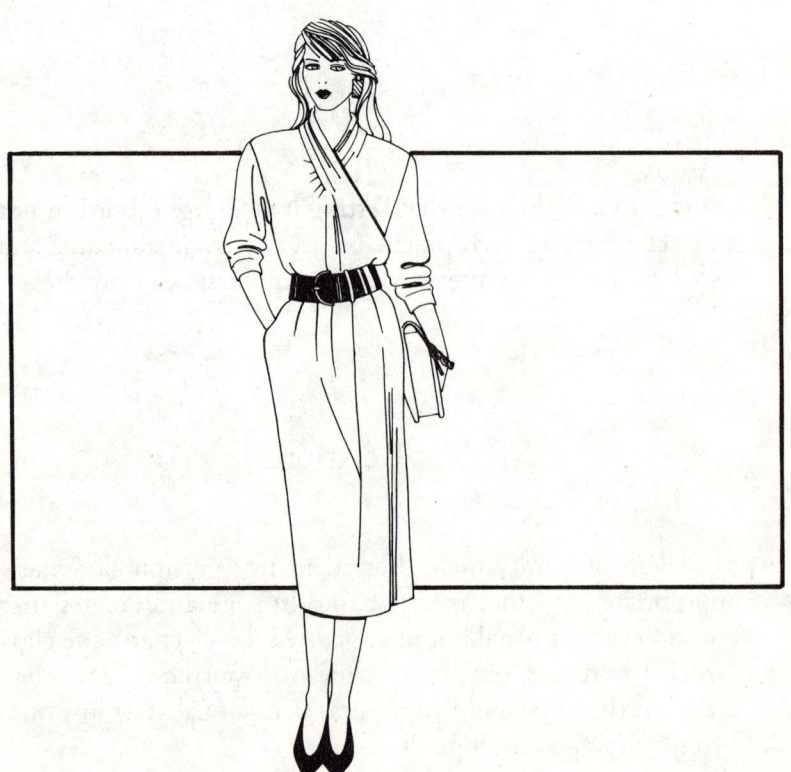

Merchandising

- "I believe a woman has to create her own identity and at the same time keep an executive appearance. A feminine appearance today is a positive factor, not a deterrent anymore."

- "I work for a dress company so I wear lots of dresses. That seems appropriate, though I don't have to do it, of course, I just do. You can't dress completely for yourself when you're in a profession. Because I work in fashion, I can wear trendy things that people in other fields can't. I'm lucky that way. The newer silhouettes are not structured anyway, though, so I believe that even in banking or brokerage houses, women can look very pulled together in terms of a soft-suit look or a jacket and dress."

- "Mix-and-match items are really perfect for work if you operate within a basic color scheme, then throw in other colors that add a new look. The right accessories can easily dress it up or make it look casual."

Real Estate

- "Real estate involves a lot of outdoor hiking around so I wear primarily jackets and sweaters. Tweed fits in well with the real estate look. I find my coat is most important because it has to be good for driving, not one of those that is too bulky to fit behind the wheel. Getting in and out of the car should be the least of your worries. Also, I wear flat comfy shoes for trekking around in muddy backyards."

- "If you talk about impressing clients, I find if I buy really quality 'country' types of garments (I love the Ralph Lauren approach), it's suitable to most situations. I don't have to look as though I'm sitting behind a desk all the time because I'm not."

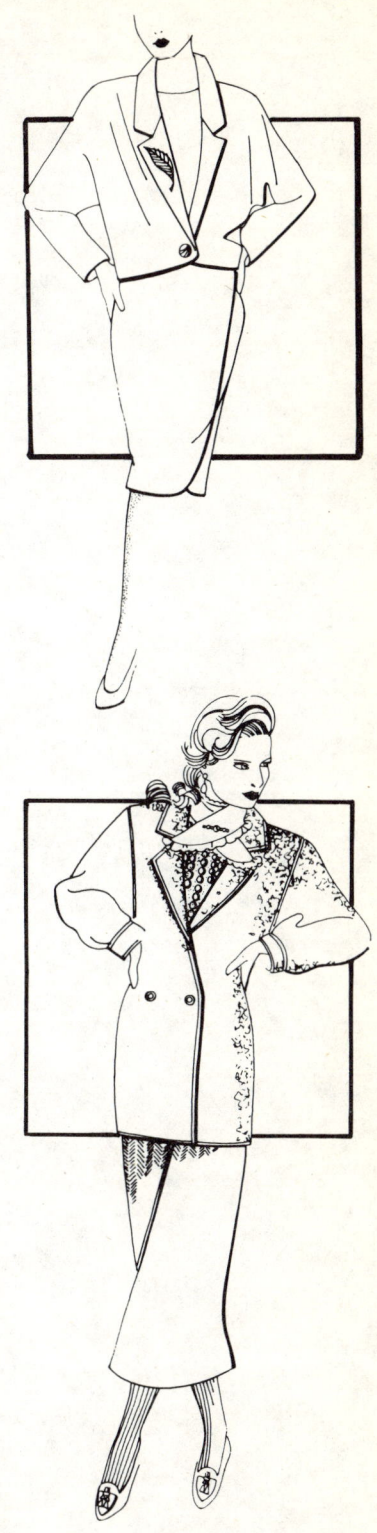

Social Services

■ "Working twelve- to fourteen-hour days is routine for me, so what I wear has to keep me from looking wilted if possible, plus it must be comfortable. In summer, I go with dresses and jackets. I need a place for my beeper and keys—most importantly—because if I lose my beeper it costs me four hundred and fifty dollars to replace it, and one dropped from my pants pocket in a blizzard last winter and was gone. So I make sure I have good, deep jacket pockets. I wear plaids or silky prints with tiny details that hide muss and wrinkles with a blazer. Sometimes I do wear slacks, a shirt and vest and blazer, all in a related color family. I go for the New York rumpled intellectual look basically, lined flannels, wools, small pinwheel corduroy—a very comfortable approach that still looks professional."

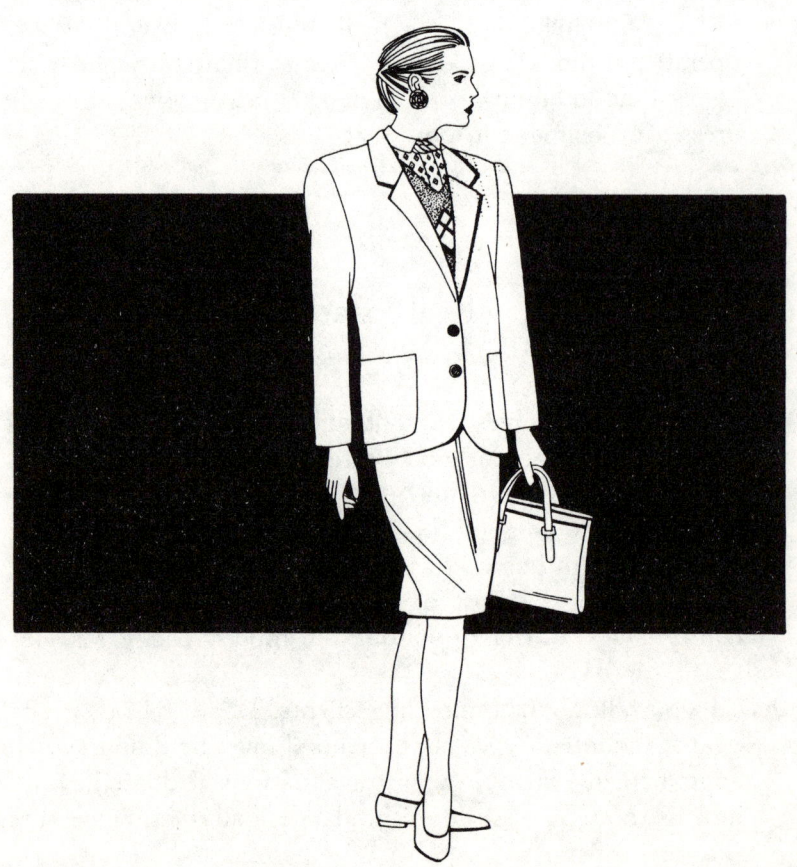

- "Mostly I walk on concrete floors at the hospital all day, so I wind up hating just about every pair of shoes I own. I am the only one in my department who doesn't wear mid-heels but goes instead for classic skimmers. I think the other women must have burned out the pain receptors in their feet. At meetings, all shoes come off though."

Teaching

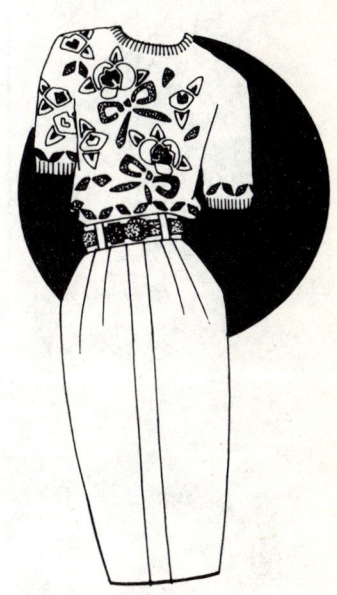

- "Working with kids, you want to capture their attention and imagination. An interesting look is a good place to start. A fun belt buckle, a patchwork jacket, unusual jewelry, bright colors, and colorful, nubby materials can do the trick. Elementary teachers have more leeway in what to wear, and many kindergarten teachers are the most unique dressers because they are trying to stimulate knowledge seeking, and they use what they wear as a way to teach. One teacher I know wears a wooden necklace with each bead carved as a different fruit."

- "Teachers in higher grades usually wear skirts and dresses. Above all, we're concerned about conveying a professional image to students who are often not that much younger than their teachers."

- "Business suits aren't really right for this setting because they convey the impression of being cool, not involved, which is the opposite of what you want. Education is the business of feelings, of establishing rapport with students. Some teachers think of themselves as teaching subject matter only, but that's not really what good teachers do."

- "We're a conservative group. My system is an upwardly mobile one. For parent/teacher meetings, I definitely dress up and may wear a suit or a tailored dress. Instead of flats I wear heeled pumps and maybe a classic pin with a scarf. Now you're presenting an objective evaluation of the child as a student and you're not talking about being 'involved.'"

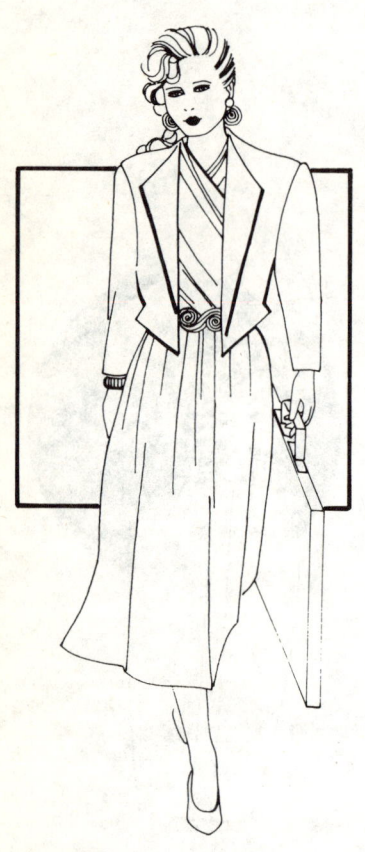

- "There's a moral stipulation for teachers in their dress, moral meaning 'upright.' That means no flesh showing, no sensuality. Feminine but not alluring. You must be morally correct, so I never wear anything sleeveless to work, no short skirts, no low necklines. You have to take sexuality out of your dress completely. You will see 'conservative dressy' and 'artsy dressy' among teachers, but never 'sexy dressy.' The last thing you want to be with students is evocative. And with a male supervisor, that's the last thing, too. You must look respectable."

Interior Design

- "I feel we can be especially individualistic when it comes to hemlines these days—some mid-calf, some bottom of the knee, but nothing shorter than mid-knee. Knits have to be

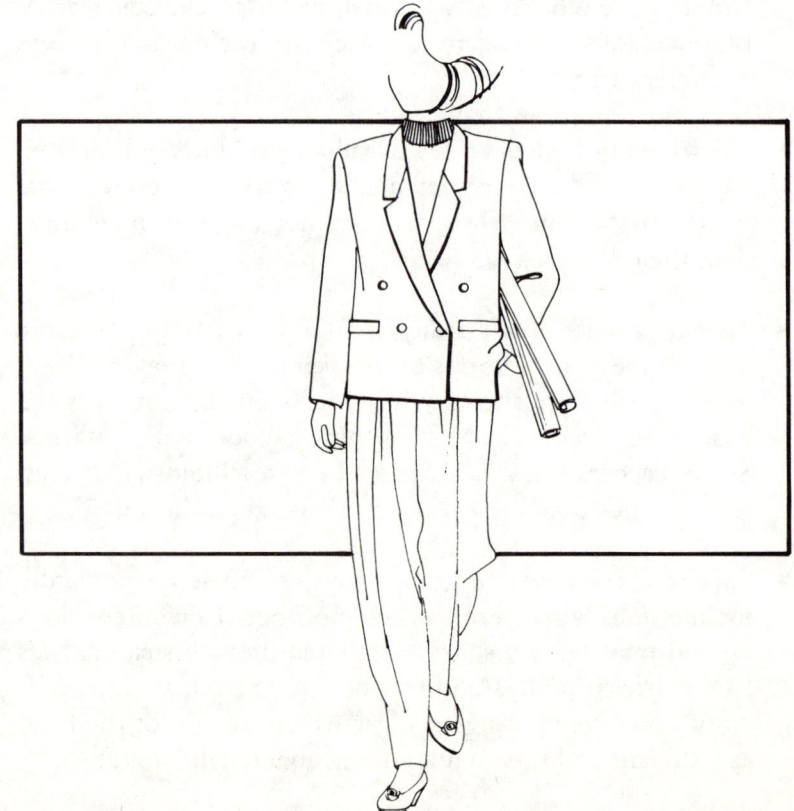

worn carefully, if at all. I don't think they make a big hit in business."

- "Right now I go for poly blends in such things as blouses. They look like silk but they can be washed. You can't perspire in silk. Just sitting in the car one day with my back touching the seat, the colors in my silk blouse faded. I don't think silk is something to be worn day after day. I believe businesswomen need garments that are easy care but still look chic."

Computer Technology

- "I like to shop boutiques because department stores overwhelm me, though I will go to them for a sale. In my field, I feel it's best to look studious, like a whiz-kid type. At the same time, I enjoy wearing things like silk jackets, long skirts because I like the feel of them. In my classes, people respond to that, too. They get bored looking at you if you're too uptight and predictable."

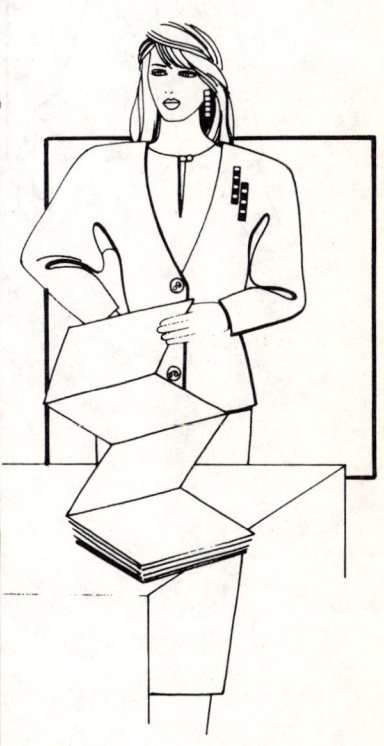

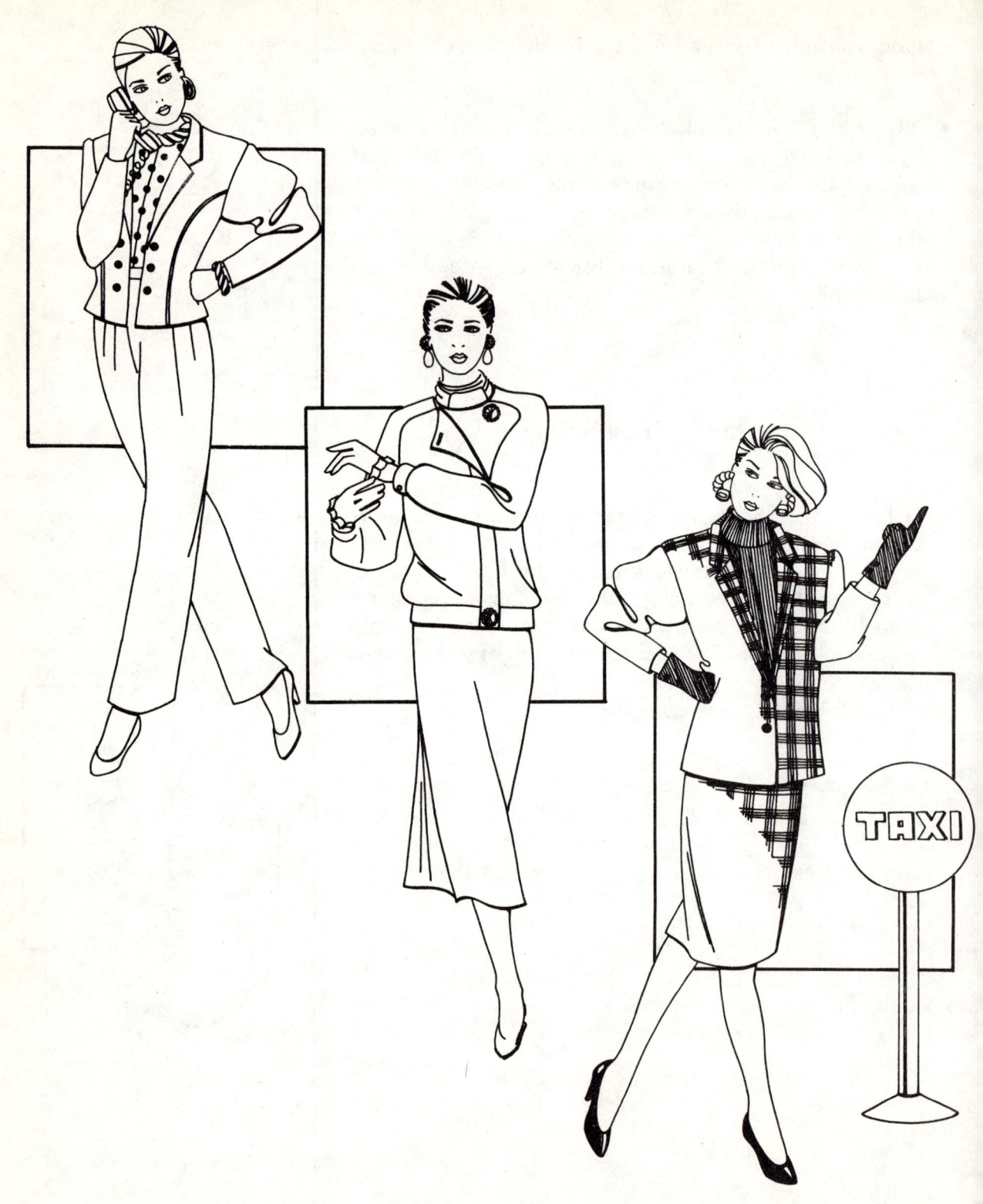

Profiles of a Soft Suit

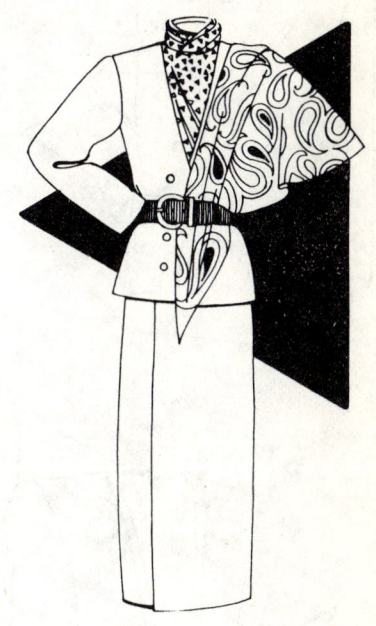

For a classic, can't-go-wrong choice for work, it's hard to beat a beautifully tailored suit. Up until recently we could barely get away with wearing anything else, and in some situations, they are still the most appropriate choice. They are also safe. It's hard to look inappropriate or out of style in a handsome suit. However, it is a simple fact that the classic suit no longer reigns supreme over the new power dressing. While a classic suit may always be an important part of the working woman's wardrobe, we no longer need to view this "ensemble" in its strictest form. A major part of the new power dressing is freedom from the confines of the hard-line business suit.

Just look around you. The "business suit" has begun to change, charged with the new spirit with which we have come to wear them. More feminine, more fun, more eclectic, the "business suit" can now be what you would like it to be.

Softer Suits

The suit is like a canvas upon which you can paint feminine

"*Not all women look good in man-tailoring. That looks good on mannish figures. If you're hourglass or full-busted, they gap in the wrong places and a suit won't do the most for you. Possibly a different kind of jacket or a tailored dress in that case would be much more flattering.*"

Susan McCone
of Jonal Boutique
in New York City

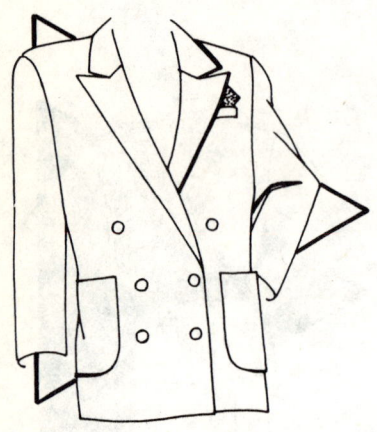

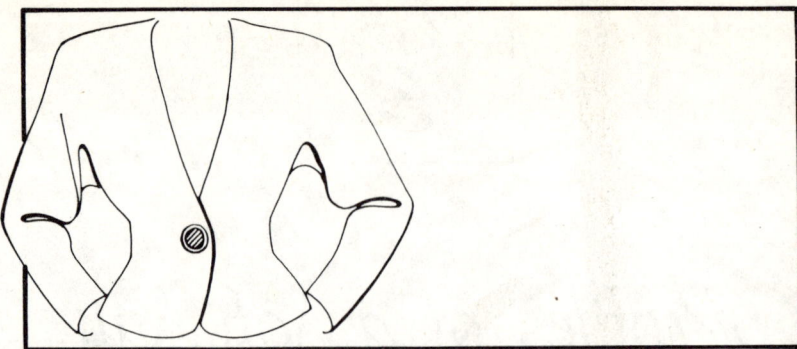

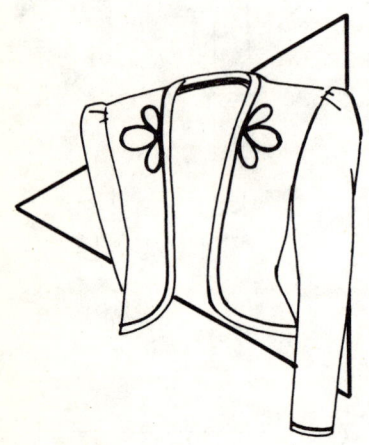

bold statements to both suit your tastes and the new power dressing. Suits used to mean one-tone, a notched collar, a straight skirt, a few nondescript buttons, and boring. Take a look at them now! No more severe, mannish lines. Suits take on details undreamed of before at the office. No longer staid, suits now make room for designer flair. Colors can be subtle to vivid. The door has opened to a whole range of fabrics as well.

Soft suiting, as the term implies, ushers in a whole new and refreshing infusion of femininity. Strict tailoring gives way to silhouette and line as major concerns. Jackets may be unconstructed, collarless, perhaps with a cardigan look or cropped short. Peplums add femininity, as does the figure-hugging cut of longer jackets which are generally much more flattering for everyone. In short, strict tailoring gives way to a curvy silhouette. (What could be more dashing than the bullfighter look?)

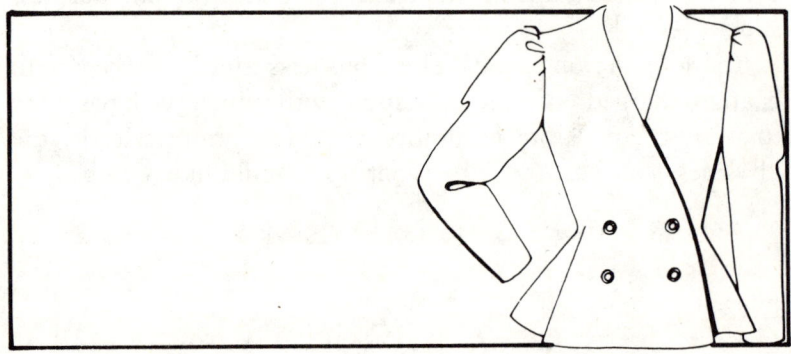

JACKETS: Jackets can be worn in varying lengths depending on what flatters the individual figure most. All lengths and shapes are more boldly "body conscious," not sexy of course, but showing off the figure more. Boxy is out. Mannish is out. The single-breasted, double-breasted basics remain an option, but when paired with the variety of collars and buttons now available, they look completely fresh and new.

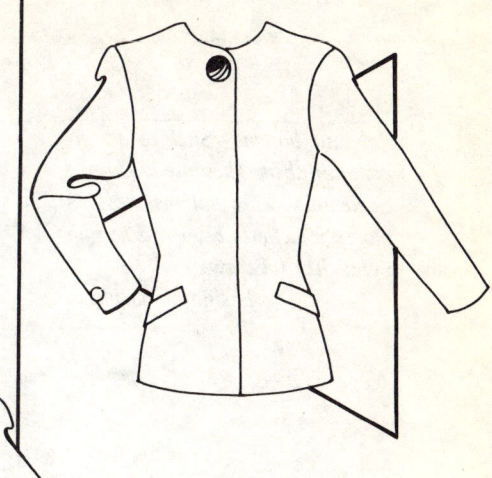

SHOULDER PADS: Shoulder pads are much more flattering when softened as they are now, rounded slightly and not quite so extreme. Believe it or not, shoulder pads convey authority and power. You'll never see a man's suit without them, and likewise a woman's suit should always have at least some shoulder padding, no matter the style.

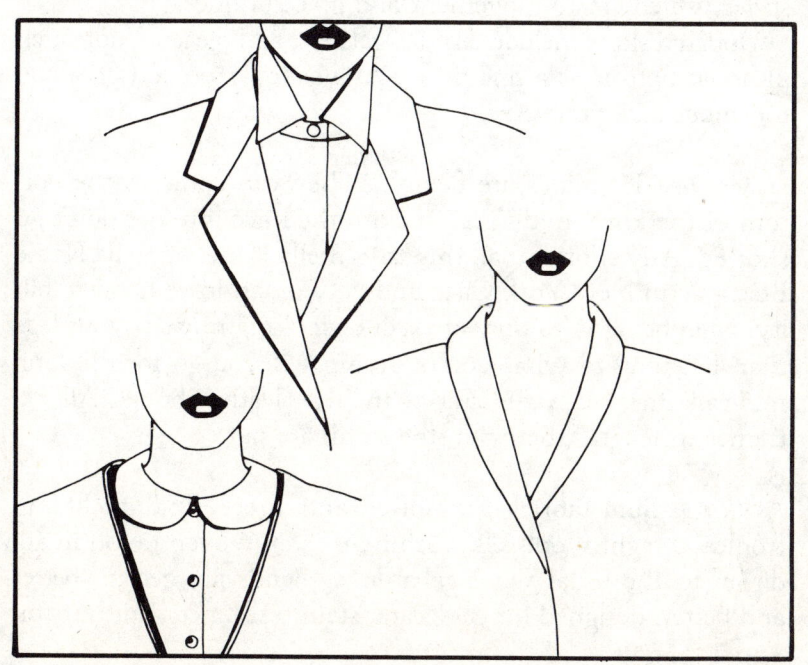

COLLARS: Collars alone come in a range of variations. There are shawl collars, collars that close high or at the top of the breastbone, at mid-clavicle, or low where the ribs join. Currently a stunning look is the *collarless* jacket. (One designer has done away with lapels, collars, *and* linings on his suits.) There

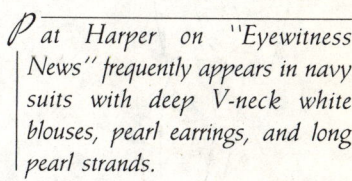

*P*at Harper on "Eyewitness News" frequently appears in navy suits with deep V-neck white blouses, pearl earrings, and long pearl strands.

43

are mock turtlenecks, shawl collars, Peter Pans, ruffled collars, tuxedo collars, wide lapels or narrow, and on and on.

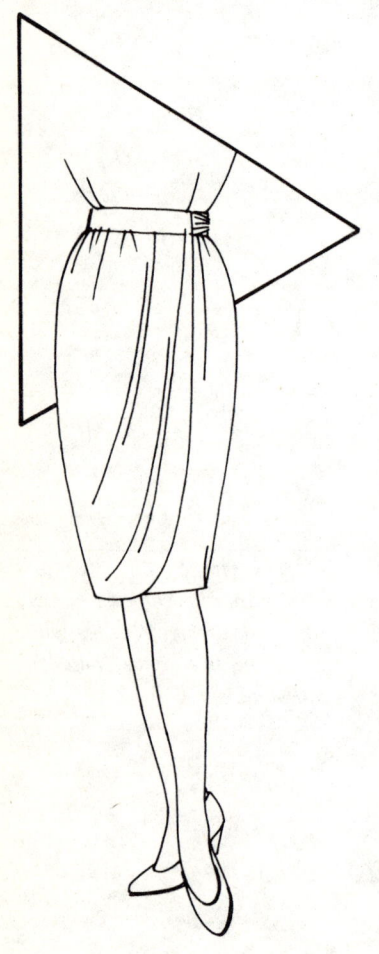

BUTTONS: Buttons now make their own bold statement. Some jackets button triangularly from shoulder to waist. Buttons are a detail to be taken seriously in suits. They can add to the overall effect, stay muted, or detract from the fine look of a garment. They might interfere with accessories, or highlight them. The right buttons can make a suit, but if they make too definite a statement of their own, they limit the possibilities of dressing the suit up or down. Some jackets get rid of those buttons in the front that never got used, and now show only a single button at the waist. Many buttons may be pretty enough to act as accessories. Generally the most economical choice is to go with simple or fabric-covered buttons so that you are then free to change the look of the suit with a change in accessories.

SKIRTS: The good news about suit skirts is that they've turned fluid. Where before they were as close to the effect of trousers as we could get, now skirts offer movement, fullness, and softness. The opening of the door to dirndls, pleats, and venetian layering has also led to draping, sarong styling, and wrapping styles which create movement and graceful lines.

Updated skirts include dirndls, gathers, and pleats. Triple kick pleats at bottom is a fine detail. A-lines look too conservative; too much like yesterday.

HEMLINES: Hemlines are flexible. They can come to the bottom of the knee, mid-knee, or skim the knee top (but don't go shorter). Any shorter than this, says Stella Flame of Stella Flame Boutique in New York City, and "a woman loses her credibility. Men being who they are will be looking more at your legs than listening to what you're saying." If you go for the long mid-calf line, team the suit with high leather boots. All extremes in length (the maxi, the mini) are out.

FABRICS: Suit fabrics are softer and more fluid including tropical-weight wool, silk, cashmere, even woven rayon in addition to the usual wool gabardine. Blends are getting better and better, designed for easy care, stain resistance and to maintain their lines. Shop carefully when considering a blend, however. A blend does not necessarily mean a bargain. The really fine ones can be quite expensive.

Look for fabrics light enough to wear in warm weather, or under a coat in winter. Include rayon and silk. Just remember that rayon is more a fabric for draping, so it will not keep a sharp line unless blended. Sheer woven wool, blends of wool and rayon, and unlined wool gabardine are all-season.

Summer: Lightweight wool is classic (beige, steel blue, gray). Cotton is casual. Silk is dressy. Linen wrinkles but is classic. Seersucker, too, is classic, looks fresh when paired with whale-size white buttons, gold jewelry, and a slim stretchy skirt.

Winter: For nine-month-a-year-wear, go with lightweight wool, gabardine or crepe, flannel, worsted wool (menswear fabric), or silk which is actually year-round. For those of you lucky enough to live in the more temperate areas, these fabrics, except for the silk, will be too heavy.

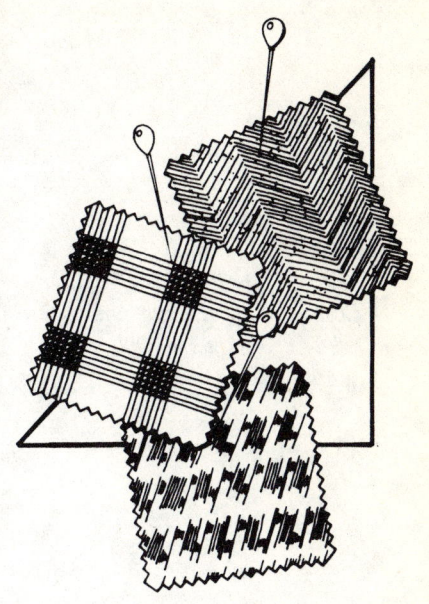

PATTERNS: Individual taste shows up in choice of fabric as well as texture and color. For instance, flecks in the fabric weave give it an entirely different appearance. Tweeds, patterns such as houndstooth, glen, or oversize plaids each project a different image. Tweeds are more casual, more country. High power is a herringbone suit which can also be matched with a black skirt. The banker's stripe even works in the more softened lines granted by these softer, lusher fabrics. The ever so slightly masculine look of stripes, glen plaid, houndstooth is feminized by showing up in softer, more feminine fabrics.

A sense of fun as well as elegance comes with small dots or larger polka dots, black-and-white checks, plaids and stripes, and paisleys. If you have your basic suit wardrobe already and want to experiment, patterned fabrics offer a wide range of choices. Some weaves mix well together, too, with suit jackets being worn with other skirts. Mixing different fabrics relies as much on experimentation as it does on a sharp eye for color and styling. (See our chapter on separates for more on how to mix and match to accomplish the mismatched suit look.)

COLORS: When buying a suit, decide on the two to three basic colors that you'd like your wardrobe to include and buy within that range. Most of us still believe that we can only wear

"I can wear a red blouse to work now. There's no need to look masculine anymore, and I don't see people doing that."
Bank Recruiter

"Personally, I don't buy anything navy because I like black better. There are different blacks as well as different navys, which most people don't realize. Blacks aren't as easy to match as one might think anyway. Know those colors that look good on you and build on that."
Charlotte J. Moore, chancellor, International Academy of Merchandise and Design

45

certain colors. However, New York City boutique owner Stella Flame reminds us, "There are so many shades to every color, that within a color there is bound to be a shade that will work on you. You don't have to limit yourself." Women come into her shop saying, "I can't wear navy, it deadens me, or beige because it washes me out." Actually, we can all wear those shades given the particular shade, proper makeup, and accessories. Learn to work with classic colors for classy results.

Classic suit colors include burgundy, teal, green, navy, black, camel, white, ivory, and gray. Big plaids can work in a suit but are limited in wearability with other items. Stick to dark colors when you choose a suit that is highly feminine. Red and teal, of course, both tend to seize attention. They are good colors to wear when giving a presentation or in any situation where you need to hold the attention of a group. Otherwise, keep suit colors subtle and bring boldness in through accessories and blouses.

Classic choices are also black-and-white prints or patterns. White with any other color looks very chic. Soften it with neutrals, tan or a gray belt or bag.

Pants Suits

Witness the rise of the pants suit. They have been around under other guises before, fallen into disrepute, and now they return as an option for businesswear. Since top designers have adopted the pants suit, their cut and style do make them a suitable choice, especially for an executive living in the harsh winter belt of this country. A beautifully tailored pants suit worn with a lush cashmere sweater and tall, high-heeled leather boots will not only feel good in 20° below zero weather, it will look absolutely appropriate in business meetings too. If you opt for a pants suit, observe the basics that apply to any suit.

Where pants suits veer off from skirted suits is in the area of large plaids, paisleys, and florals, none of which belong with pants. Styles can't help but appear more mannish, especially when they come in pinstripes, glen plaids, or houndstooth. Yet some of the beautiful designer pants suits come in these fabrics. Counterbalance the severity simply by accessorizing. Wear a luxurious heavy-silk blouse, gold link chain bracelets, large-scale gold earrings, and otherwise elegant, feminine accessories to counteract this effect. Besides jewelry—earrings, necklaces, or bracelets, a flower pin would also grace a pants suit nicely. Playing against the man-tailored feeling is an exciting fashion technique.

NOTE: The very last thing you would want to wear with a pants suit is a tie, so don't even consider it!

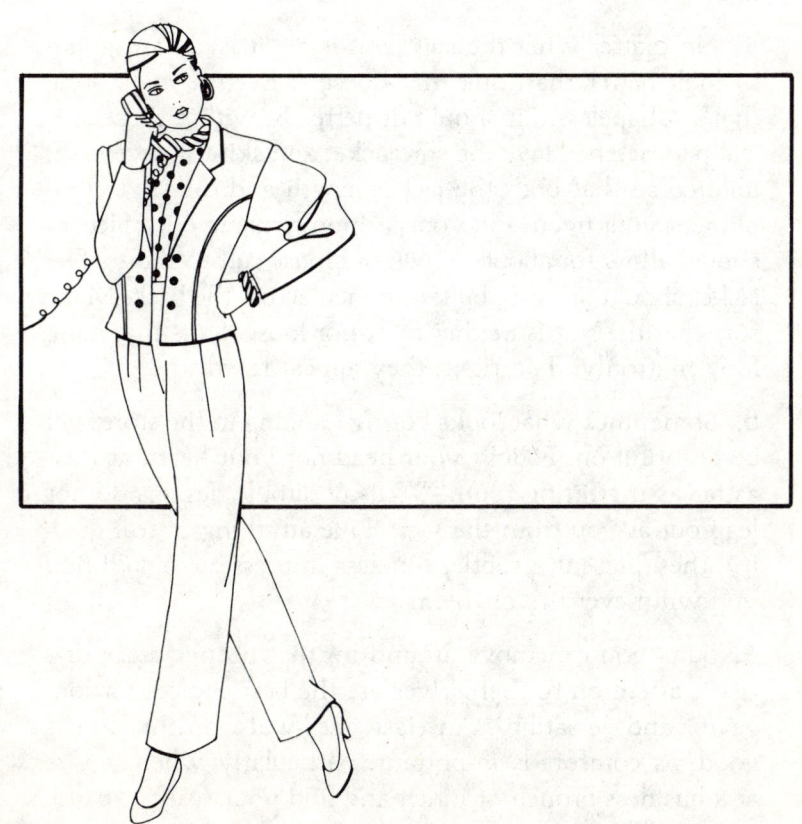

"A soft draped neckline for a blouse makes it more dressy."
Management Consultant

How to Choose
Your Own Soft Suit

1. Go for quality. Buy the best suit you can afford.

2. Choose neutral colors in a suit such as black, brown, beige, ivory, navy, or gray. A teal or a cranberry suit is fine if you already have several in classic shades. What you're aiming for is colors that will work with various shades of accessories in order to get the most wear in many situations.

3. Keep unusual designs to a minimum. If you already own several neutral-toned, quality suits, you might want to buy one that includes an up-to-date silhouette with perhaps a more extreme cut in the jacket. Still it is easier to change the look of a simple suit than it is an extraordinary one.

4. No matter what the suit is, if it fits it is always going to look better than one that doesn't. Even if it's a style that's "shapeless," it should fit perfectly within those special perimeters. Have the suit jacket and skirt, if necessary, tailored so that both the jacket length and the skirt compliment your figure and your fashion requirements. Sleeves should allow for about 1/4-inch of blouse cuff to show. The jacket should not gap, bulk or bunch across the back. Make sure that the suit is neither tight nor loose. Suits that hang look matronly. Too tight, they appear tawdry.

5. Sometimes what looks boring hanging in the store will be beautiful on. Follow your head not your heart, at least as far as the fitting room. Well-cut simple designs do not leap out at you from the rack. Like anything of real quality, they present a subtle, timeless impression. You'll find you will never tire of them.

6. Suits you can move around in, that do not draw dramatic attention to themselves are the best choices for longevity and versatility. An elasticized-waist on the skirt is good, as comfort is important, particularly when you're at a business brunch or lunch and find your waist expanding as you eat.

7. Jacket shapes and colors should complement other skirts in your closet for the ultimate in mixing-and-matching wearability. This also makes business travel packing a breeze. One suit paired with several exchangeable skirts makes up a week's wardrobe.

Accessorize the Soft Suit

ACCESSORIES: Accessories play a dominant role in soft suiting. For example, full, floppy silk flower pins replace the stark bow tie, a day many women thought would never come. Jewelry has risen to the occasion by assuming much greater visibility. No longer must we adhere to severe standards which ruled out everything but pindot diamond earrings or a short, minimalist strand of pearls. Accessories keep pace with the revolution in the world of business fashion.

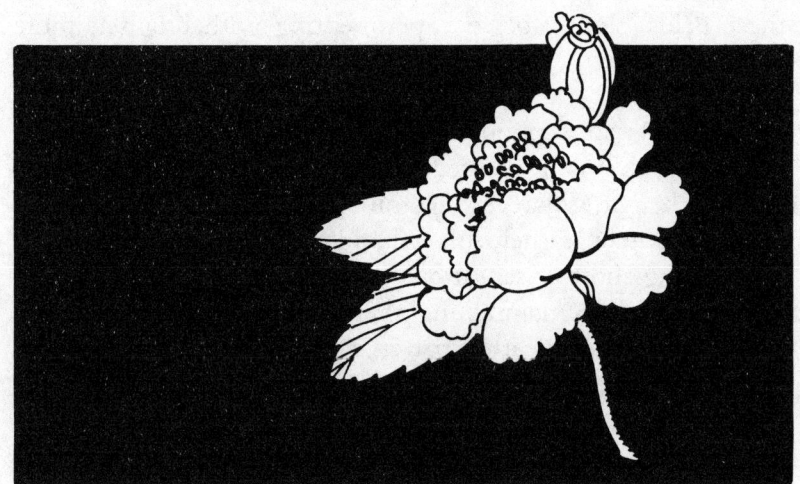

BLOUSES: Luxury blouses work like a charm in such fabrics as crepe de chine and charmeuse, or anything in cashmere or silk. It is also possible to get an effective look with simple, flat knits, lightweight jersey, cotton, rayon, silk with just about any kind

"*The key is simplicity. You have to be able to wear a suit on all different occasions. A black linen suit, well cut, with a French silk flower pin to dress it up, maybe black and crystal beads, constitutes a really beautiful look. In this case, black-and-white beads would go too much with the basic colors, be too obvious and wouldn't work.*"

Boutique owner
Misook Kim,
New York City

Independent movie producer Sherry Lansing wears crepe suits, preferably over black blouses.

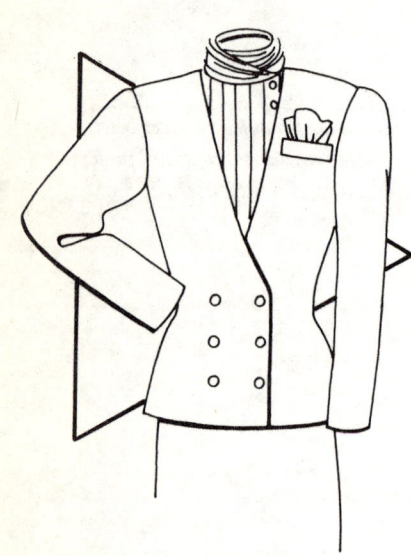

of neckline, shawl or notched collar blouses in rayon/silk or linen. All work beautifully with suits.

Natural fabrics look the best. However, some polyester blends can barely be distinguished from silk except when it comes to washing care (poly washes and drips dry). These updated polys aren't cheap and don't look it either.

Lacy blouses are fine so long as they aren't see-through. Avoid any blouse, no matter the color, that is sheer enough to show the outline of a bra underneath.

Go for details such as pleating, touches of lace, and interesting collars. Collars that work especially well with suits: jewel necklines, no collars, double-wrapped collars, crushed-neck collars, simple V-lines, embroidered placket fronts, notched collars, shawl collars, and tuxedo collars.

It's fine for blouse colors to make a bold statement. Hot colors such as chartreuse or fuchsia update a suit instantly. Pick colors that highlight your complexion so that you don't look haggard when you're tired from working overtime, but stay away from metallic colors or Day-Glo types of flashy prints.

Blue and white used to be the accounting uniform colors for blouses. No more. Navy suits with pale-blue blouses also used to be uniform colors for sales execs. If you work in one of these fields, slowly begin experimenting with brighter, more flattering colors.

SHOES: Suits are supported best by the medium-heeled power pump, but that is not so tedious as it sounds. Heels can run a range of height, whatever is comfortable yet dressy; they might be suede, patent leather, soft Italian leather; and the colors now are nothing short of sensational.

Pumps, while maintaining their classic status, come with subtle designs and leather patterns now, and so offer yet another area to make an individual selection. Lightning-like zigzags of contrasting colors bolt along the sides of some otherwise sedate shoes. Lizard-patterned leather insets at the toe and heel make an otherwise plain soft leather pump into a selection that shows real taste.

Besides this cornucopia of shoe possibilities, we can now also change the look of a classically simple pump with bows or flowers or ruffles that clip on, which makes a shoe more versatile than it's ever been before.

BELTS: Do wear a belt with a suit. Most suits look under-dressed without them. Cool belts for summer are made out of woven leather or tailored straw. A wide belt should be two to three inches at most. If you're overweight, select a narrower belt.

Look for textures such as faux ostrich or crocodile. Woven leather or mixes of textured leather, rope, or canvas also work well. Light tones make good summer choices. For winter, one brown and one good black belt is all you need.

GLOVES: Try textured crochet or soft leather or suede gloves in glowing shades to set off a suit. Gloves offer another op-portunity to add a bright color to your basic suit tones. Fuchsia or chartreuse, pinks, teals, and reds all spark up a business look, especially when shoes match.

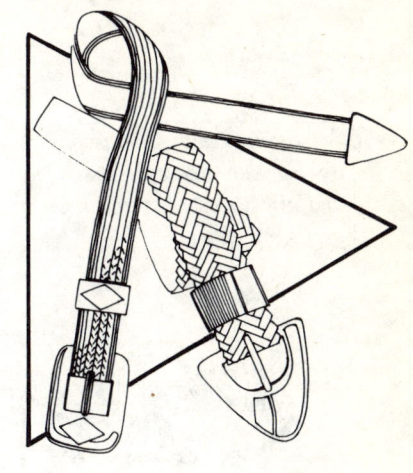

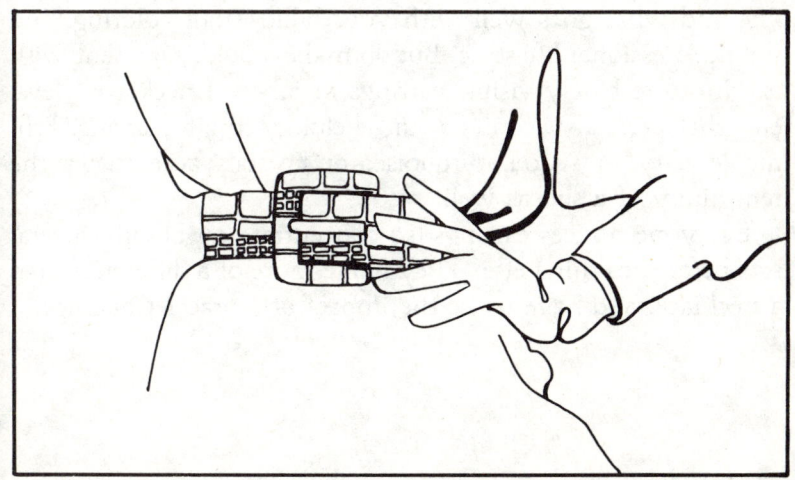

SCARVES: The right scarf choice can set off a suit; the wrong choice can ruin the look of it. Scarves should be expensive, running anywhere from forty to 400 dollars. Expect to keep them for a lifetime. Wrap at the waist, neck, head, hair, drape over the shoulder, or wear as a shawl over a suit on those days when the weather is just a nip too chilly for a suit alone. Scarf clips are new, and stickpins can be used to keep a stole in place.

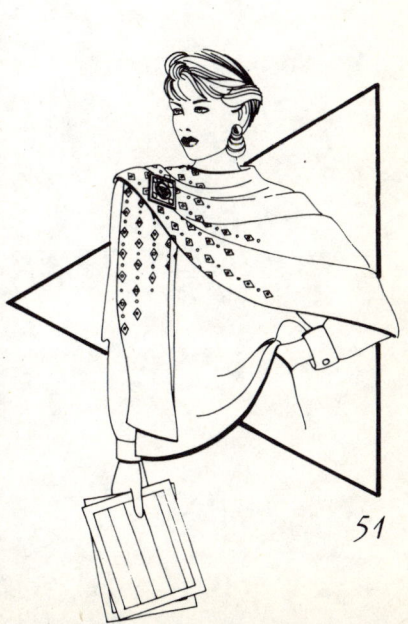

51

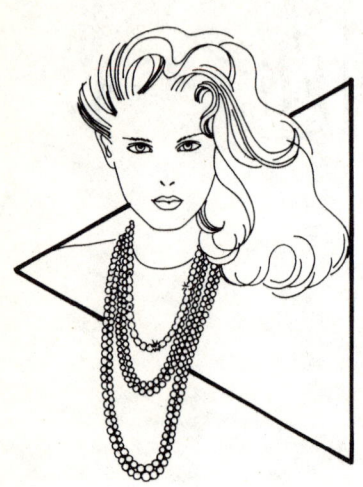

TV reporter Carol Jenkins pushes up her suit sleeves occasionally and also wears rows and rows of pearls.

JEWELRY: Jewelry, along with everything else in executive women's fashions, explodes with boldness. That single strand of pearls has become ropes and ropes of colored crystal beads, gold chains, or pearls. Earrings are huge and clunky, either in gold or silver, and often with a colored stone. On some occasions, you might even want to wear something glittery or dramatic, such as dangling earrings holding a huge pearl. The more exotic and quirky the jewelry the better, so those items picked up on foreign travels, such as ceramic pins and antique brooches, should now be exhumed from the drawer and worn. You will find they perfectly highlight feminine wear and individuality.

Good costume jewelry, the kind that costs anywhere from fifty dollars up, is the thing to shop for. You don't need many pieces. Perhaps one to two necklaces, several sets of earrings, and a few bracelets will do. Gold jewelry doesn't have to be real gold to look smashing. Try on all jewelry before buying; it will look different on you than in the case. Buy what you like and what goes well with your build, your coloring, and your professional life-style. But do make a bold statement with it. No more barely visible earrings or ethereal necklaces. Jewelry that perfectly accents a suit is clunky, bright, strong. Ethnic jewelry in wood, turquoise, or crystals accentuates the femininity of a suit as well.

Everyone notices earrings, so concentrate on buying several sets before anything else. They make more of a difference than a necklace, and have twice the impact of a bracelet or rings.

Three Types

With a working knowledge of basic lines, current styles, and your own professional dress codes, it is now time to get creative. Following are some suggestions within three basic fashion categories: Classic with a Twist, Avant-Garde, and Exotic. Use these outfits the same way you use window and floor displays, to stimulate your own imagination, to help you better envision

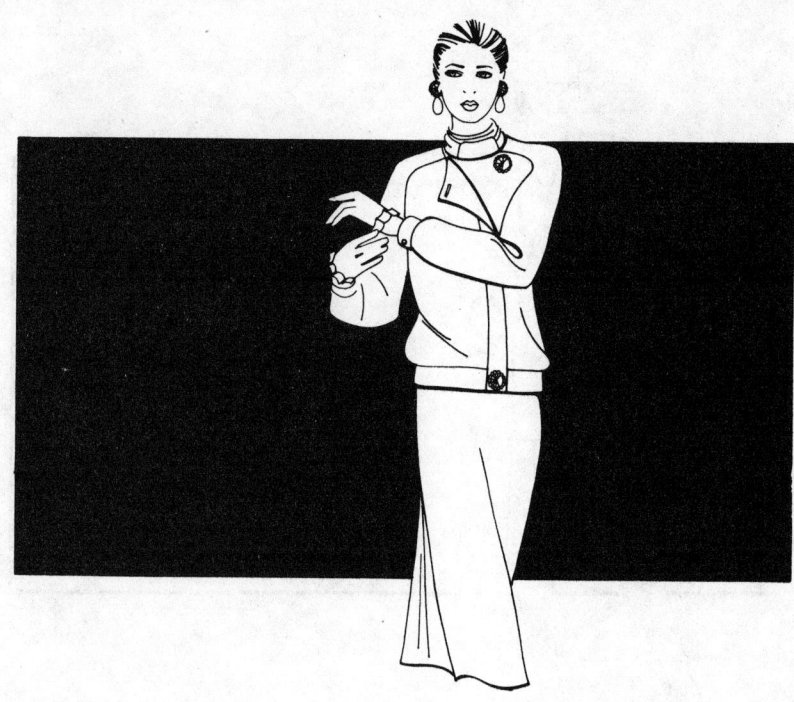

combinations as you shop and to bring forward items from your wardrobe that you might not have thought to use in this manner before.

Classic with a Twist

- A creamy turtleneck with a wide gold-buckle belted suit.

- A blue crepe suit with a dropped waistline, a sparkling button closing at the waist, a slim skirt, and sparkling earrings.

- Red on red. A red suit with a red V-neck, possibly a wrap blouse with deep-red gloves, red shoes, and a large red silk flower pin.

- A red suit with a pink paisley silk blouse and gold earrings.

- A bankers' navy pin-striped long-length suit with a satin-striped high-neck blouse and a navy newsboy cap.

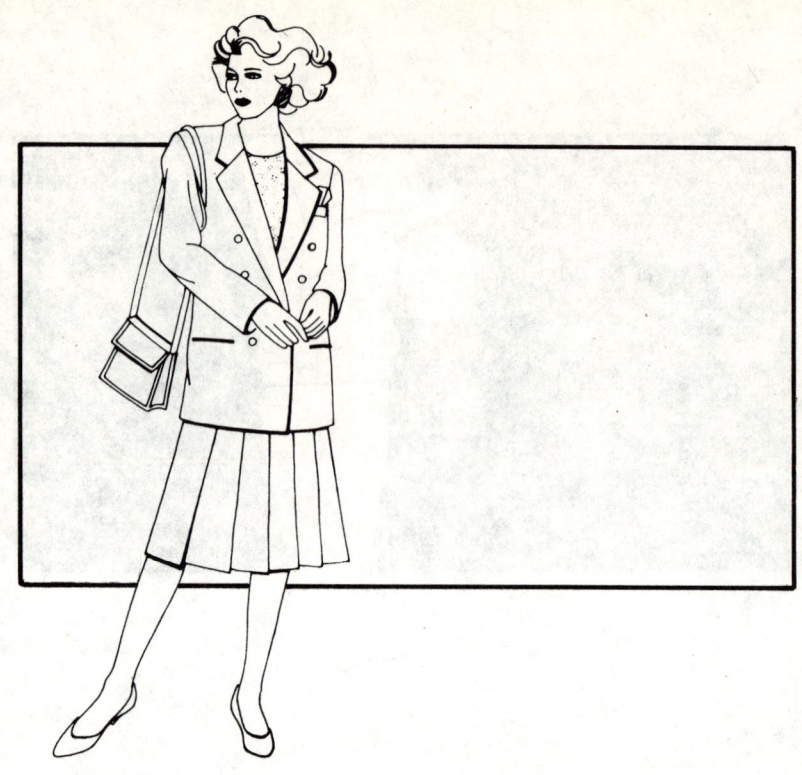

- An all-black suit with silver buttons if possible, silver earrings, and red gloves.

- To update a charcoal flannel double-breasted suit, hem the skirt to just skimming the knee, add a many-wrapped scarf at the neck, brown woven leather power pumps, and a luggage-toned bag.

- With a deep-rose suit, wear a pale-pink blouse and shoes, and pale-pink-toned hose. Drape a scarf over one shoulder.

- A peplum-jacketed suit over dirndl skirt, an oversize shawl in metallic colors that pick up the suit color, such as purple with red and yellow.

- A white long-jacketed suit, preferably with a knife-pleated skirt, add gold accessories, and purple gloves or a purple bag.

- Add gold buttons and a wide belt with a gold buckle to a navy pindot suit. Wear with a cream wrap jersey blouse.

- With a linen collarless jacket over a flared skirt, wear thick strands of choker pearls.

- A houndstooth suit in black and white goes well with a pink blouse, gold chains, and a gold lapel pin.

- A gray glen plaid notched-collar suit? Wear with a black jersey turtleneck, huge gold hoop earrings, and black leather gloves.

- Plum is so chic today, especially when it's combined with purple, red, or even blue. Add a blue paisley silk blouse, plum pumps, a plum/blue shoe clip at the neck.

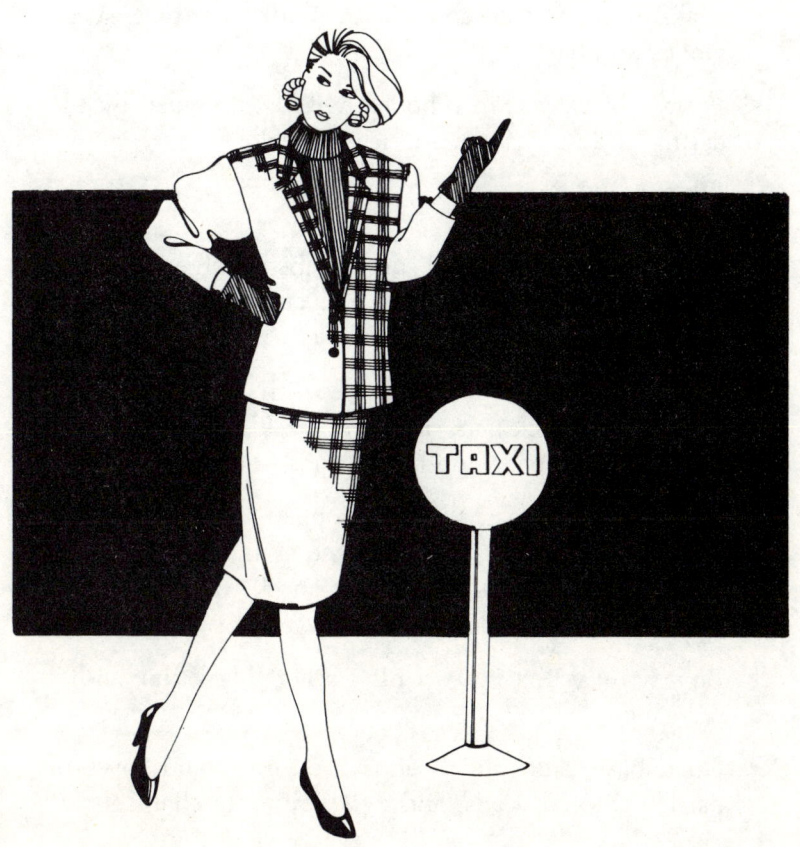

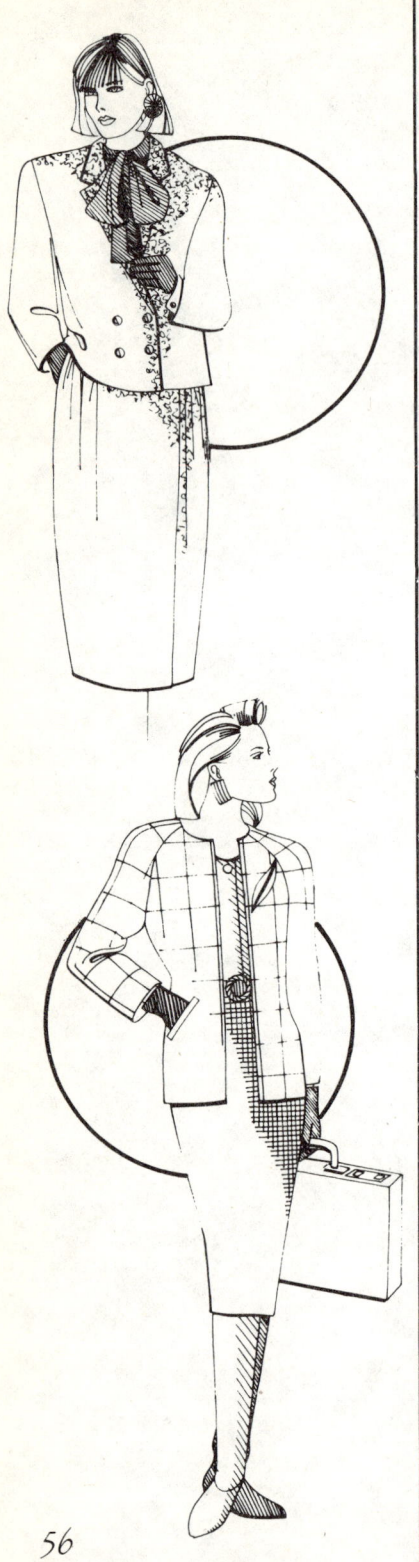

- Keep the executive spirit by teaming a black-and-white checked suit with a red and black paisley scarf, a tiny red silk floral pocket square, and a huge antique Rolex watch.

- A double-breasted tweed teamed with a crisp white high-collar blouse, huge floppy black crepe neck bow, a wide black belt, red/gold earrings, and black gloves will give a slightly British flair to a chic pulled-together look.

- A white wool crepe collarless suit will look terrific with black gloves, a black faux lizard bag, and a scarlet floppy silk flower pin.

- A black and white houndstooth suit jacket worn with a slim black skirt, a gray cashmere pullover, and a cream silk scarf.

- Make a navy suit come alive with light-blue suede gloves and hat.

- A staid black suit in a boucle weave is rescued by the daring of a low, square-neck white blouse.

Avant-Garde

- A red-and-black checked suit matched with a red jersey blouse, red belt and gloves, red earrings, black-toned hose, and high black leather boots.

- A lavender suit looks fantastic with a black bow or neck clip, a black belt, open slingback *pink* heels, and a self scarf wrapped round and round—no blouse.

- A red double-breasted bolero cropped jacket with black buttons and a matching slim-line skirt teamed with a black-and-ice striped mock turtleneck, black/gold earrings, black-toned hose, and black power pumps.

- Be a wow when you set off a severe black suit with a red cape.

- To a basic suit, add a choker or rows and rows of paisley colored beads, and a paisley wool challis stole.

- A green and red plaid suit teams with a silver clunky necklace and silver drop earrings.

- A shaped suit in plaid—remove the buttons and the collar. Hold it shut with a wide belt, and underneath, a tuxedo-style white silk blouse, and huge stand-out white pearl earrings.

- A startling blue double-breasted suit, nipped at waist, with a slim-line skirt, matching gloves, and a bright-*red* turtleneck jersey blouse. Gold hoop earrings, a gold bracelet, and red power pumps.

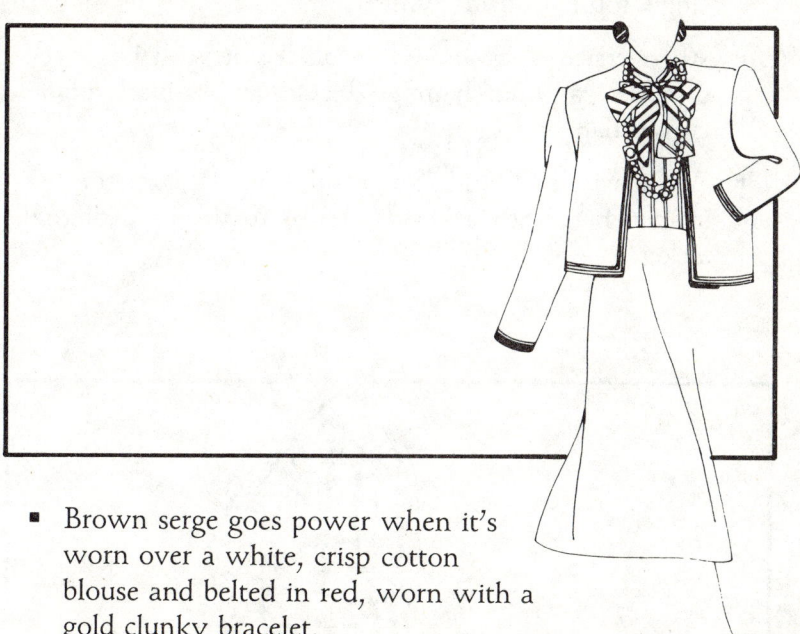

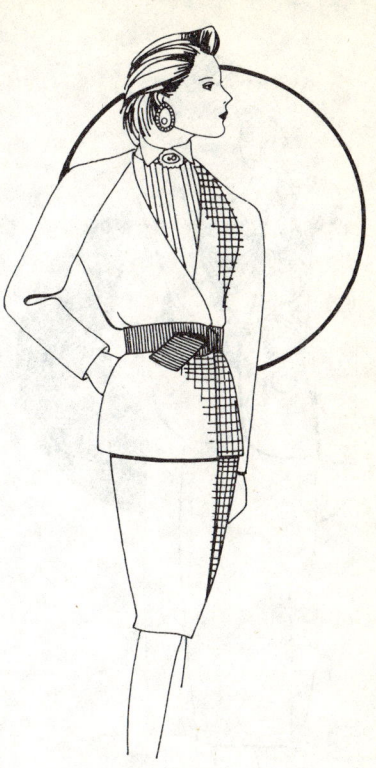

- Brown serge goes power when it's worn over a white, crisp cotton blouse and belted in red, worn with a gold clunky bracelet.

- A plum wool suit with a black silk ruffle-neck blouse, a wide black belt, and a floppy silk flower pin in teal/plum.

- A cranberry knit cardigan suit zooms up to stratosphere level with the addition of a black-and-cranberry striped blouse with a self-tie collar, a wide gold chain necklace, and black/gold clunky oval earrings.

- A houndstooth cropped jacket with a matching skirt can look outrageous with a cream blouse, a shawl in

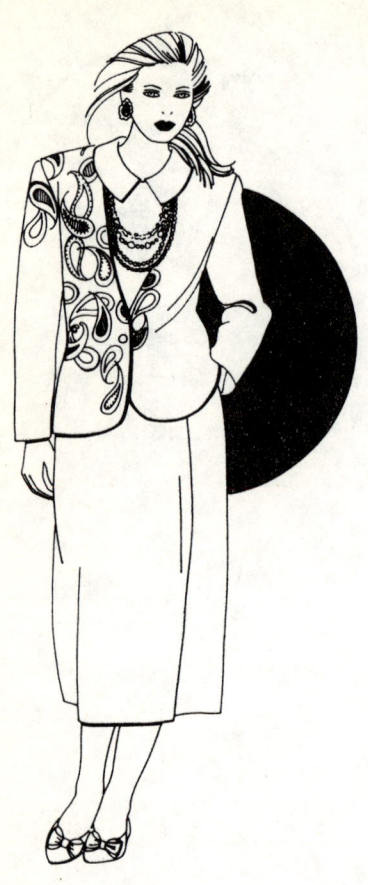

black, gold and red worn around the shoulders, a wide black suede belt, a black quilted bag, and gold earrings.

- A paisley jacket with a black or wine skirt, many strands of colored crystal beads, wine-toned hose, and bowed shoes.

Exotic

- Pink on pink: A short jacket, a slim pink skirt, a pink high-neck blouse, and pale-beige hose and shoes.

- A red suit with a slim black belt, black gloves, and a single top button in—white!

- An oversize black-and-white plaid suit with black accessories, a three-chain gold belt, and a black high-crown hat.

- A fuchsia suit and black-and-fuchsia geometrically shaped hat, with a bow fastened to the back of the jacket.

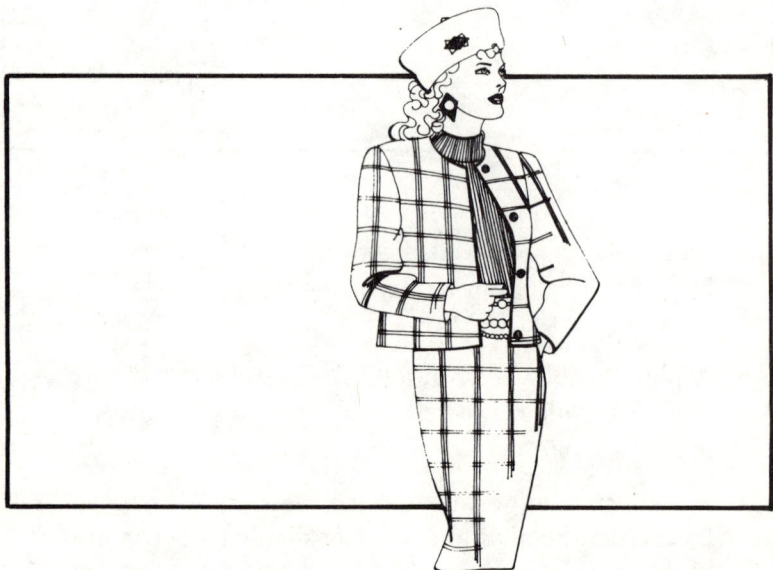

- With a blue suit, a black-and-white leopard print oversize silk scarf tied cowboy style (point forward). A red jersey turtleneck blouse.

- A windowpane plaid suit matched with a satin handbag, and a papier-mâché necklace of roses.

- A shawl of vivid stripes worn over a man-checked suit.

- A charcoal fitted jacket with a slim skirt and a single gold closure at the neck becomes exotic with a black jewel-neck silk blouse, black/gold loop earrings, black-toned hose, and black power pumps.

- A black-and-plum paisley fitted collarless jacket with black rosette clip-on buttons, and wide silver Spanish fan-style earrings.

- An extra long-line single-breasted black-and-white wool checked jacket with a black-and-white striped scarf, and a red and black paisley blouse.

- A mink-colored cropped jacket with calf-length slim skirt, brown gloves, brown-toned hose and brown skimmers, and chartreuse silk pocket pouchette.

- A double-breasted navy suit with a violet lace blouse, a purple bowler with a peacock feather, and purple gloves.

- A purple plaid suit with a deep-purple shirt, pale-blue suede shoes and matching gloves, blue hoop earrings with a ceramic loop necklace.

- A fiesta black linen bolero with a slim skirt. Wear with a tropical floral silk blouse, bright gloves, and a silver Spanish pin.

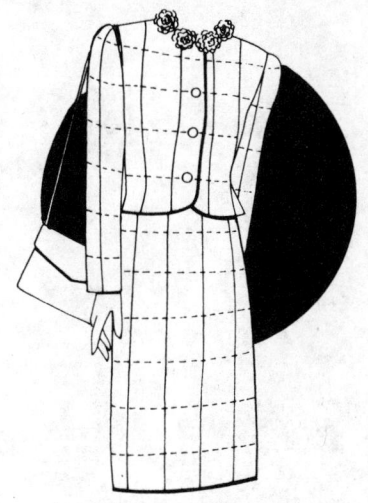

Dos and Don'ts

Do

Include textures and patterns when considering buying a suit, such as boucle weave (thick), glen plaid, or herringbone stripe. All add interest.

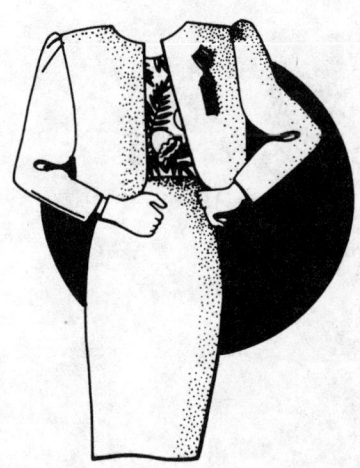

Update your current suits by having a tailor restyle the notched collar of an old suit jacket into a collarless line.

Check yourself from the back when trying on a suit. Make sure it doesn't bunch at the shoulder blades or buckle at the neck. When wearing a suit, be sure that your slip doesn't show out of a slit.

Add a belt with an unusual buckle for a newer, more chic look.

Accessorize according to your size as well as professional style.

Try a long jacket over a short skirt, and checks over a dotted blouse. In other words, don't be afraid to be contrary.

Wear just a scarf at the neck in summer—and no blouse—for a dramatically chic effect. Clip in place with an antique pin.

Create an entirely new look by adding something special such as an elaborate antique brooch or a breast pocket fuchsia silk pocket pouchette (scarf).

Don't

Wear a neckline low or skirt slit high, and do not wear skirts above the knee, unless your assets allow, and even then only slightly above.

Make your suit a tight squeeze.

Go for flowery or overly ruffled suits.

Cling to oversize shoulders (they overpower).

Wear anything extremely puckered, ruffled, or bowed.

Wear anything initialed, even if they are famous initials. The only possible exception is a tailor-made shirt with your initials on the sleeve cuffs or breast pocket.

Wear inexpensive suit fabrics such as cotton broadcloth, polyesters (in anything but a silk or wool blend blouse), and no knits.

Wear short-sleeved suits or low necklines.

Choose bright colors in the basic suit unless you cool the effect with an accompanying blouse and accessories in white or icy tones.

Go overboard on accessories. Generally, the busier the suit fabric, the fewer the accessories should be.

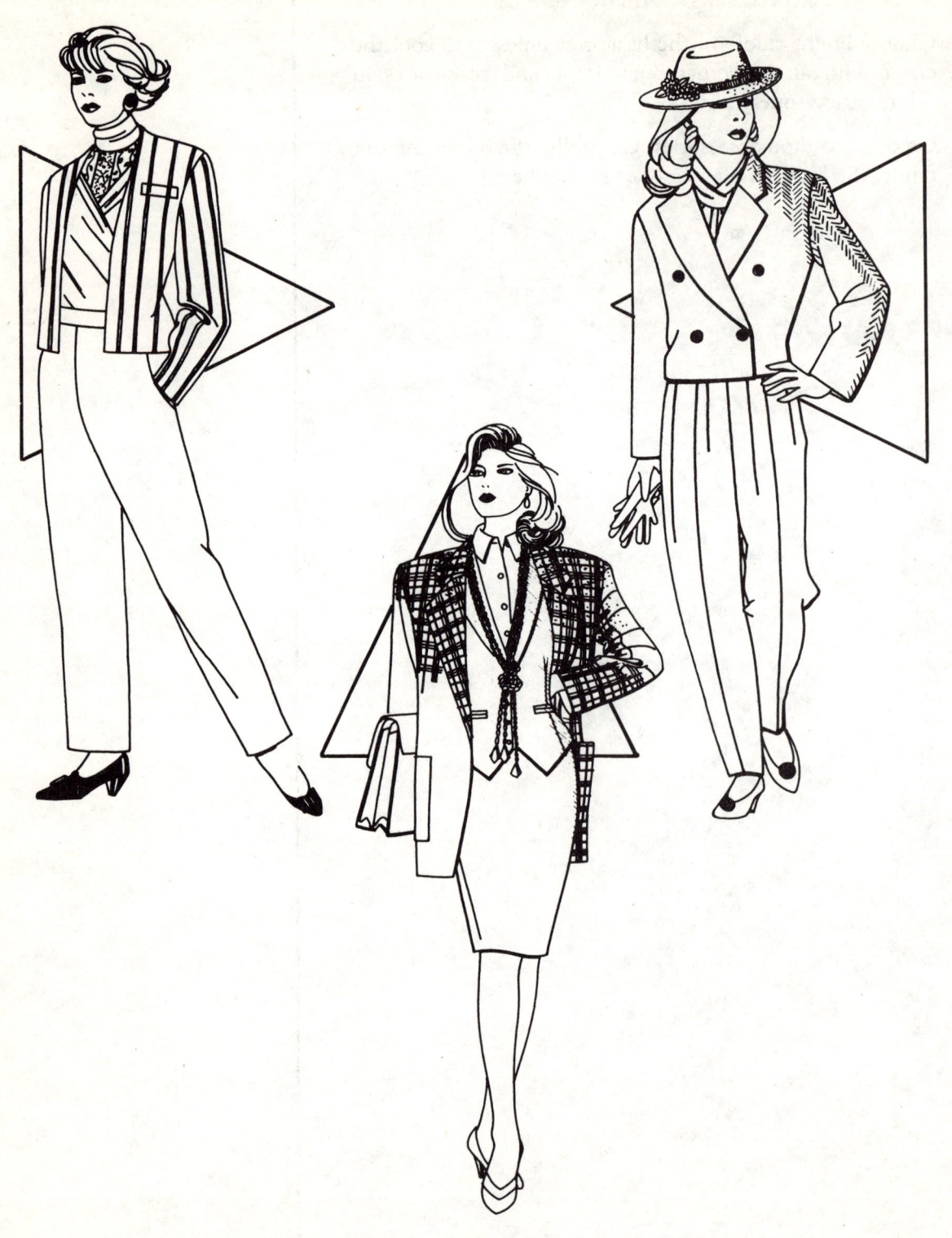

CHAPTER 4

Separates But Together

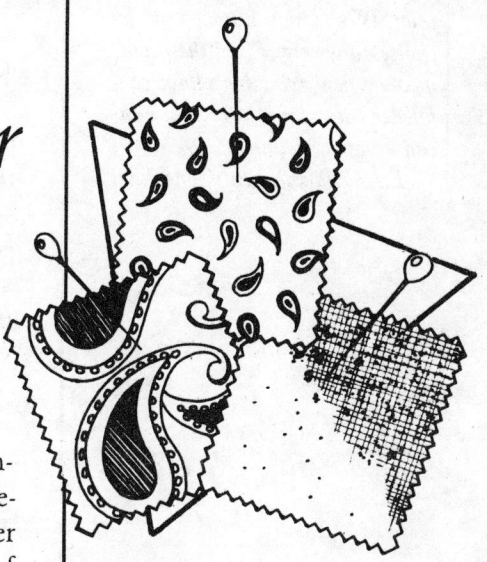

Separates include skirts, blouses, sweaters, blazers, and individual jackets for an "unmatched suit" effect that requires a more skillful hand at pulling the look together than do suits. Separates are probably either the bane of your fashion existence or the joy of it. Few of us are in-between on the subject. That's because it isn't easy at first to coordinate those disparate items. Almost everyone has to learn how to choose one skirt that will go with another jacket with yet another blouse or sweater and then handbag, hose, gloves, hat, jewelry. Every piece should work together as one to achieve real career chic. European women are famous for this skill born of economic necessity. They have had to learn to create variety out of a few garments and still look striking every time. Here in this country, we are only just beginning to do this, as women start to regard their clothes as long-term investments.

What lies at the root of most of our mix-and-match confusion is the lack of important basic fashion information: We don't know what we like, and we don't know what looks good on us. If we were savvy about these key points, we could experiment with mixing and matching and never go far astray.

The best way to learn is by studying magazines, other people, shop windows, and by asking questions; then trying things on in front of a mirror alone or with a friend. The more you experiment, the easier the process becomes, and the more confidence builds.

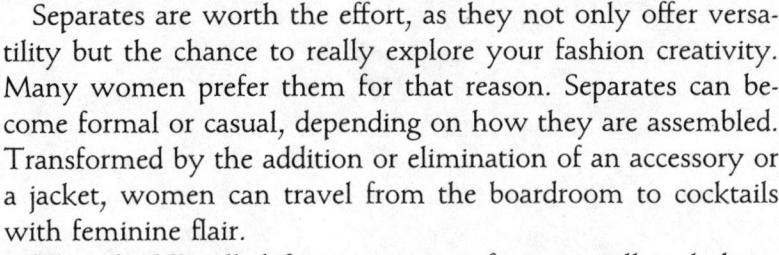
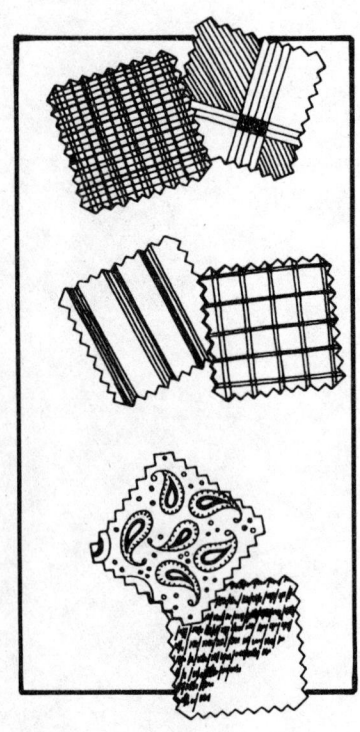

Separates are worth the effort, as they not only offer versatility but the chance to really explore your fashion creativity. Many women prefer them for that reason. Separates can become formal or casual, depending on how they are assembled. Transformed by the addition or elimination of an accessory or a jacket, women can travel from the boardroom to cocktails with feminine flair.

The "look" called for in most professions still includes a jacket, so when you think of separates, at least for right now, think of a skirt, a jacket, and a blouse or, in some instances, a sweater. However, though a blouse or sweater with a skirt (no jacket) used to be a no-no—a throwback to school days—skirts, sweaters, and blouses are being upgraded to the point where, if they're handsome enough, they can certainly be worn to many offices without any repercussions.

The Unmatched Suit

Putting a blazer or jacket, perhaps a suit jacket, with a skirt of another fabric, pattern, or color basically constitutes the "unmatched suit," the current power look. Tomorrow's business styles will have more to do with dresses. But for now, the teaming of disparate fabrics, colors, and prints makes the most up-to-date fashion statement.

Department stores are keenly aware of the call for unmatched suits and stock them already put together, which results in buying a suit that doesn't technically match. Racks now contain solid-toned and plaid jackets, skirts of differing weaves, and even solid and printed blouses that work together. The garments are being shipped in capsule groups which suggest to the customer how to put things together since most women do not have the time to run from rack to rack or try to remember what they have at home and what they saw at another place. This will help you in beginning, but as you grow more confident you won't want to automatically accept these packaged ideas. Your own personal fashion fundamentals will empower you to take new and flattering chances.

To achieve a sense of the polished effect that makes the

unmatched suit work, study how certain plaids almost inexplicably blend with dissimilar ones. Or a check with a stripe, or a paisley with a houndstooth. Look through fashion magazines and browse in boutiques. What you find may be more appropriate for some businesses than others, but it will give you a sense of what melds and what does not. In a way, it's similar to cultivating an artist's eye. Relate what you see to what makes *you* comfortable and happy to wear. Then experiment with accent colors to tie the unmatched suit together.

Balance and proportion are crucial in coordinating the unmatched suit, so remember not to overdo. Women who are short or overweight need to be wary of cutting themselves in half with vividly contrasting colors. One way around this is to work with contrasting fabrics rather than color, and subtle differences in patterns, rather than, say, a yellow jacket and a purple skirt.

Don't become a fashion victim. Keep in mind that less is often more. For example, if you're stuck in the black mode—black skirt, black jacket, boring blouse—instead of overdoing on jewelry or even a bright blouse while holding fast to the solid black line, substitute a short fuchsia houndstooth satin-backed jacket and wear it over your black blouse and skirt. Add a black bow or a black flower to the jacket. Try a simple pair of gold-toned earrings and stop there. No more jewelry, no necklace, no bracelets. A single separate item such as this bright houndstooth jacket needs very little in the way of accessories.

Jackets

You should have at least one classic blazer, and probably will now want to include one short jacket for fuller skirts. A waist-cropped jacket can take gathers or dirndling. A longer jacket looks better with a slim-line skirt. Buy within your three-color strategy to make life easier those mornings when you rush to dress for the office.

Jackets as part of the unmatched suit must look neat, and that means, among other things, that jackets should end where

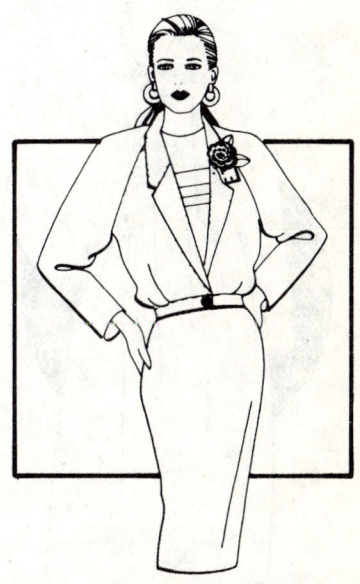

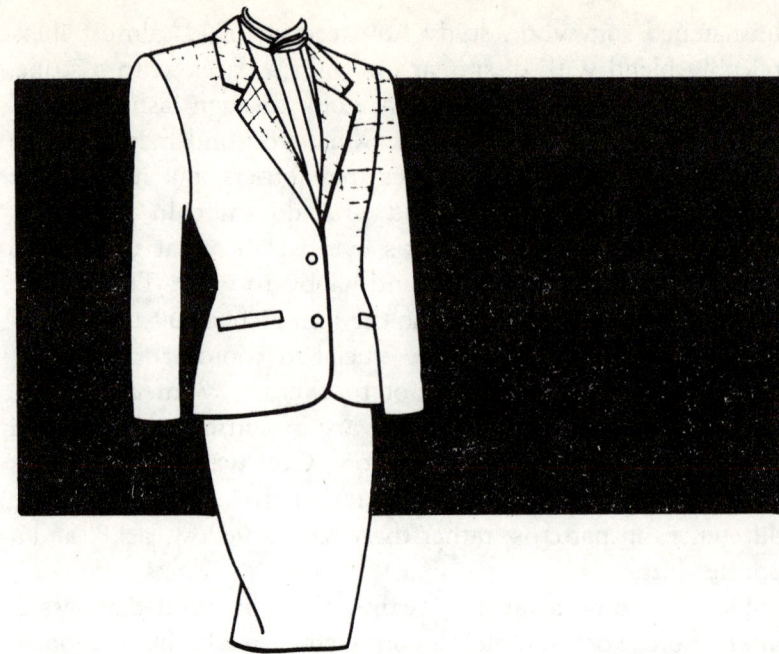

"*Calvin Klein came out with skirts too short for me, so I took a black gabardine suit I adore that had gotten shiny, took it to a dressmaker who copied it except making the A-line skirt a slim line, and that's how I got a black skirt to wear as a basic with different mix-and-match jackets. It's sort of my own version of Calvin Klein.*"

Jewelry Store Owner

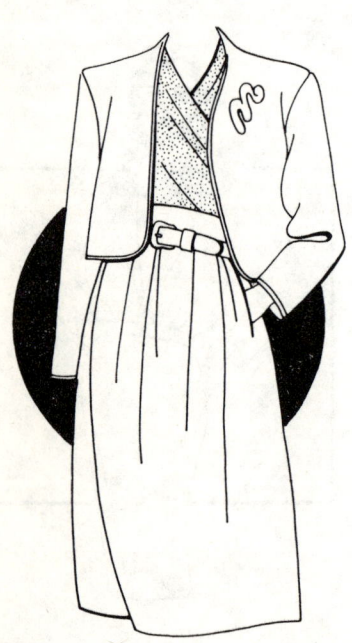

they are supposed to. If it's a short jacket, it should just cover the waistband. If it's long line, it should hit below the hips. Where a jacket should end depends on both the style of the jacket and what looks best on you.

Jackets should have pockets, preferably unobtrusive ones such as slash pockets, which provide that much important place to put your hands but do not take away from accessories by stealing attention. Keep to color basics: two neutral and perhaps one fashion color or pattern. All three colors should coordinate with the rest of your wardrobe, of course.

Skirts

The classics that seem as though they have always been with us and which somehow never become outmoded are pleats, A-lines, dirndls [full or modified], and slim-lines with or without slits or pleats. Variations available to choose from include venetian-blind layers, side pleats, bottom pleats, sarong and wraps, and even tulip lines. A high waist can be very chic if you have a long, slim torso. Skirts today are either soft and fluid or figure-revealing slim. Either way they emphasize femininity.

Again in skirts, the wise fashion buyer looks first for neutral colors in tones that coordinate with her jacket wardrobes. Skirts can incorporate a bit more color and flair than jackets, reflecting chic plaids and paisleys. However, they should still be chosen with an eye toward an interesting coordination with at least several jackets.

Skirts, like suits and jackets, should be made of fine fabrics such as lightweight wools, silk, flannel, cashmere, or a good blend. The best ones are lined, well cut and complimentary to your jacket styles. If you're looking to coordinate a particular skirt, take it with you when picking out a jacket.

Blouses

Blouses open up the new power-dressing door to an explosion of colors, details, fabrics, and style. Here is where you heighten the effect of your femininity and individuality, and give yourself the variety you need to make sure your soft suit or unmatched suit looks completely different from when you wore it three days ago. The importance of a good blouse cannot be underestimated.

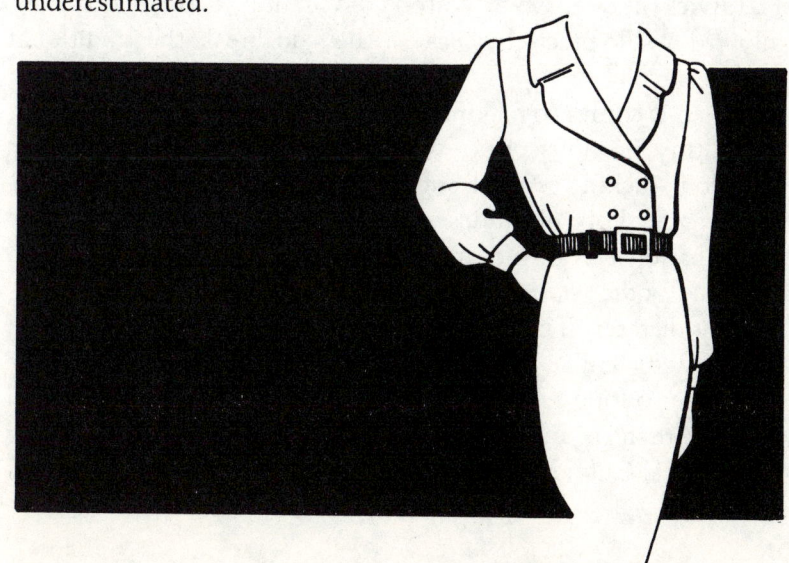

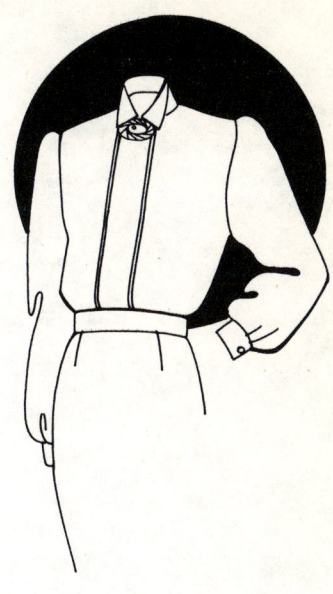

There's always the "Cagney and Lacey" look: a kind of "Miami Vice" chic on a budget—tweedy jackets with V-neck sweaters, open-collared blouses with blue and gray herringbone, or yellow on yellow with earrings for a more feminine effect.

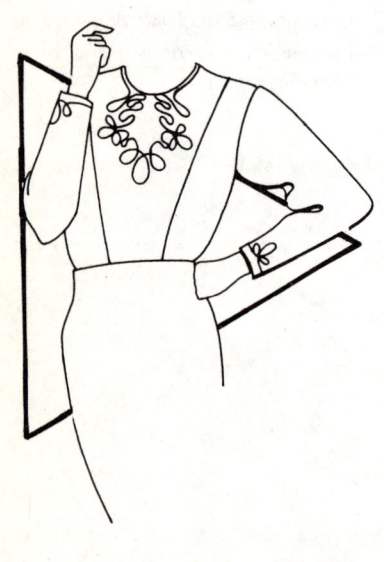

Most businesswomen today prefer silk, and for good reason. There is nothing like the effect silk gives. It looks expensive, feminine, and beautiful all at the same time. Silks come in all colors, too. In fact, the only drawback to silk is its care. Silk needs dry cleaning or, with great care and cold water, handwashing and light ironing. Many women just don't have the time for the handwashing, and dry cleaning can get very expensive if you find yourself having to clean a blouse after one day's wear.

An alternative to silk is either a silk/poly blend or 100% polyester, which must be carefully chosen. Most polyesters are not going to look great, but some more expensive poly blouses can barely be distinguished from silk. What's more, they drip dry. There's nothing like a poly blouse for a business trip, but even for the office, an expensive polyester blouse can be a very real option. For a feminine yet tailored effect, poly/crepe de chine makes for a silky look in classic lines, even in a notched collar with a hidden button placket and button cuffs. It's machine washable, too.

Satin does not fit into an office setting, but it can be worn with just the right outfit for a business dinner so long as it is tailored and not elaborate. No see-through blouses such as organza, handkerchief linen, or voile.

Then there is cotton. Stripes both wide and narrow fit the cotton background and can be worn very well with an unmatched suit. Cotton gives a clean, crisp look that is quite different from the lusciousness of soft silk. Designer Cathy Hardwick likes to wear cottons, switching to them occasionally from silk precisely because they do break the traditional look.

When it comes to picking out a good cotton blouse for work, avoid tiny precious prints which are boring and tend to look like flour sacking. Avoid button-down collars which spell minor league. Lots of ruffles generally don't work, but on the other hand, if you find an expensive cotton blouse, awash in a ruffled bodice and sleeves, Spanish style, go with it. Again, quality dictates. Tuxedo pleats are good. A high collar is fine, and a wing collar can be fun. Any kind of soft neckline is feminine so long as it doesn't show a lot of flesh. Pale jacquard stripes are nice and provide a lovely backdrop for stunning accessories. Cuffs requiring cuff links are more formal than button cuffs, although you might choose to go with a button cuff to avoid an over-jeweled effect.

Some updating blouse details are soft full sleeves, dropped yoke, and shawl collars. Antique lace collars on a blouse make it special. Avoid puffed little-girl sleeves, sheer-lace or nylon knit. No deep, revealing necklines. No sweatshirt or tee-shirt looks. If you have a traditional but boring shirt, huge buttons can relieve its severity and save it from the give-away pile.

Embroidery down the front of a shirt can be too obvious, but if beautifully (and not overly) done, it could be just the touch that causes an unmatched suit to look like one of a kind. Embroidery on one collar tip might be stunning. A white blouse with a front panel of white embroidery giving a white-on-white effect is quite feminine and pretty. A graceful wide fichet collar has a somewhat Puritan look which also goes very well with jackets.

In summer, a wide-sleeved white shirt with a pleated peplum for belting works effectively over a slim skirt. Also in summer, a lightweight tank or sleeveless shell *can* be worn *underneath* a lightweight jacket, but the jacket should not be taken off at the office, as going sleeveless looks too casual—and revealing.

Keep at least one white and one cream blouse in your wardrobe. Include one or two solid colors and a patterned blouse to spark up an unmatched suit. Accent colors should be bright like fuchsia, chartreuse, rose, yellow, and grassy green. Nothing updates an outfit like a hot color.

Sweaters

The main thing to remember when wearing sweaters is: Make sure they are not suggestive or revealing; This depends mainly on how they fit. Sweaters tend to fit snugly and this creates a voluptuous effect that does not blend well in the business environment. That's why until now sweaters have been avoided by most businesswomen. However, there is no reason why the new fashion freedom can't include a carefully chosen sweater that fits loosely but is also in a weave with a more flattering, tighter finish than most soft yarns.

Diane Sawyer of ABC Network News wears sweaters occasionally, and accessorizes with simple jewelry such as colored earrings, gold necklaces, and sometimes a scarf around the waist or neck. A lot of silk whites.

"*The mistakes I see other execs making is that clothes are too revealing, don't fit properly, or aren't suitable to the occasion. I'm amazed at how some people will show up for a luncheon in just a skirt and blouse.*"
  Casting Director

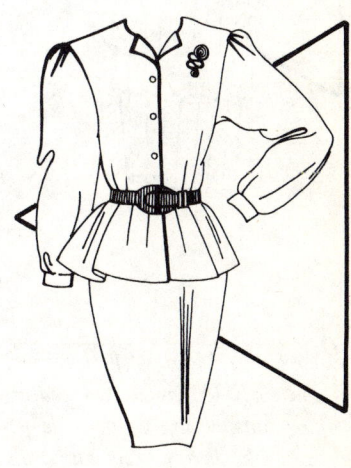

69

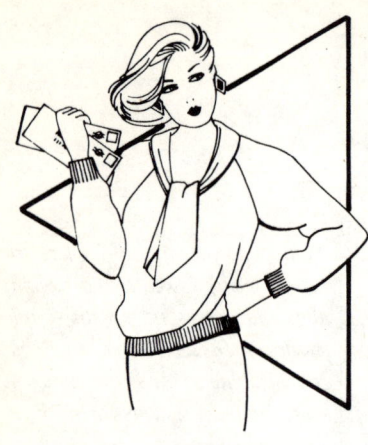

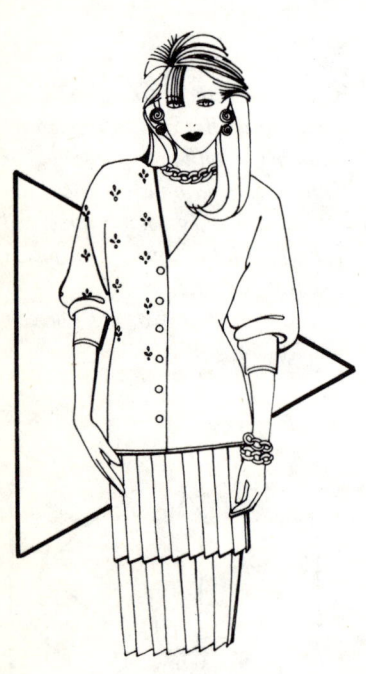

To wear a sweater as a blouse it should be of lightweight wool or cotton and of fine weave. That way it can also be worn under a suit or unmatched suit without being too warm. Nothing sets off a suit better than a classy cream lamb's wool sweater with a detail like a teardrop collar. Carry through on the cream in gloves and hose and prove everyone wrong who said you couldn't wear a sweater to work.

Sweaters have a softening effect that blouses cannot achieve. A white sweater with some angora and a band hem as opposed to ribbing, and band cuffs, can be worn over a skirt—with or without a jacket. It might also be belted. A heavy gold necklace with gold loop earrings stand out like rare gems on the backdrop of a soft, classic sweater.

Should you wear a black sweater with beaded trim, even a slight amount? This is an item that could well be bought and saved in the office closet for a business dinner. Substitute the daytime blouse and jacket with the beaded black sweater, wearing it either with a slim black or red skirt, or a skirt that blossoms out into pleats a foot from the hemline. For accessories, wear a clunky silver bracelet and perhaps silver earrings, depending on the amount of ornamentation on the sweater.

A crewneck sweater with rhinestone button detail can be worn beautifully with a suit or a cashmere/wool/silk wrap or pencil-slim skirt. A wool jersey blouse (a compromise between a sweater and blouse) with either a shawl collar, turtleneck, or drape neckline is another variation of sweater that can easily go into most executive suites with aplomb. Fine wool-knit turtlenecks or a wool and rayon turtleneck in frost colors are other possibilities, as is a wool/rayon cropped, front-button sweater with a business collar which could be worn with a skirt—no jacket—and belted. A burgundy cashmere or soft white sweater in an overblouse style should also be belted and worn without a jacket.

Cardigan styles in a tight weave create a suit effect when paired with the right skirt, such as a gray sweater with a gray plaid tiered skirt.

One very feminine, elegant look which is acceptable in certain business bastions is a luxurious white lamb's wool sweater with flowing full sleeves teamed with a white wool skirt and silver earrings. This is a perfect winter business look in a field such as advertising, design, or administration.

Pants

The way to wear pants in the workplace is with a jacket, either as a pants suit or an unmatched pants suit. They might also be coordinated with a classy bolero sweater. Today's pants come with pleats, or soft lines. They're wide, and they're high-rise. A lot of them come in pinstripes or fresh checks. The shape is soft, with wide legs, and they look particularly smashing with a short-cropped jacket.

Pants depend greatly on tailoring and proportion. They offer another choice to skirts, particularly in winter. A pair of charcoal wool soft-draped pants with a wide-shouldered checked jacket can look very chic. Again, whether this type of outfit proves suitable depends on the profession. An unmatched pants suit—or a pants suit of any kind—may be too relaxed for many offices.

Accessories

Look for timelessness in accessories. Keep them simple, uncomplicated. Go for obvious quality such as classic silver, gold, or pearl in classic shapes, and clean lines. Avoid the overly ornate or dramatic, and look for quality of construction. Work with a small core of accessories that you like and show your originality in those few items.

ACCENTS: When adding accent colors such as a pocket square, or gloves, or an enameled bracelet, think in dots, stripes, patterns, and vivid colors. Striped racing gloves can certainly jazz up an outfit.

Vests are a very good way to change a look by adding a color underneath the jacket. Silk or knit, these are an addition that can carry with them a great deal of personality.

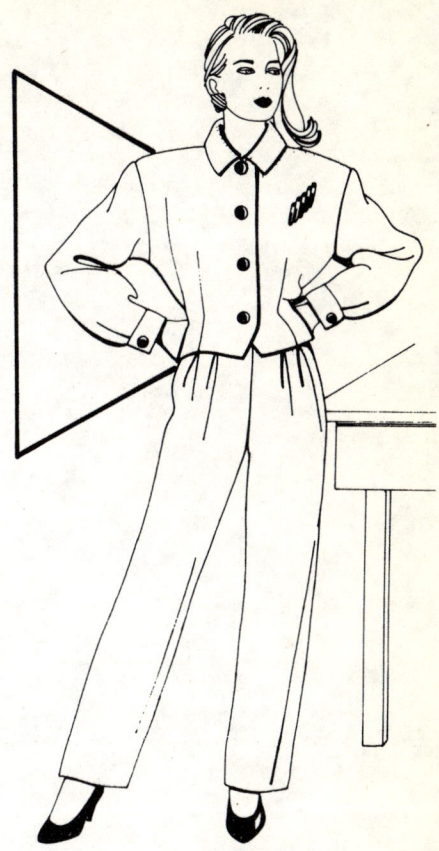

"*Pants are okay for some, but I'd say in a power-job situation, or a male-oriented office, I would stick with skirts.*"

Office Manager

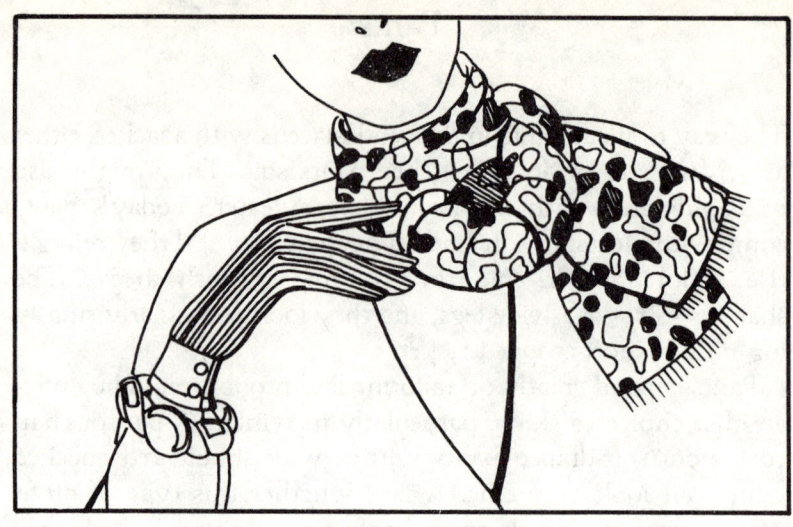

BAGS: Bags should not be oversize. Make sure you can easily find things in them, such as your pen and paper or business cards. What you carry inside should be handsome, too, such as your eyeglass case and credit-card holder. Do not carry a clutch purse.

BELTS: No cheap plastic belts with a good skirt or pants. You must look solid, reliable, and exquisitely feminine. Nothing informal, dramatic, sloppy, inexpensive, poorly fitting, mannish, extreme, unimaginative, or too dressed up will do.

HAIR: Don't forget accessories also work in the hair, such things as combs, barrettes (careful here, though, no little-girl looks allowed), enameled barrettes, headbands (also very iffy), flowers, and bows.

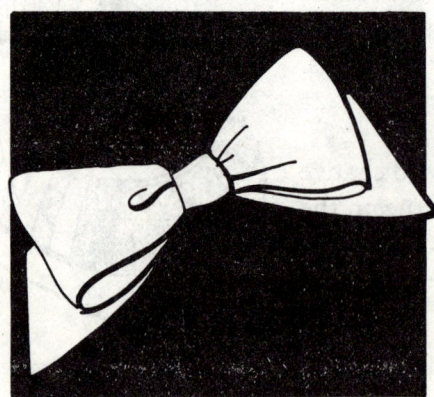

SHOES: The whole range of footwear comes into play with separates, from medium-heeled pumps, boots (both tall and ankle height), to low-heeled skimmers. Wear flat shoes with skirts and blouses or sweaters; heels with the unmatched suit; boots with pants. Then break these rules, too. A low ankle boot in a smashing new shade would be quite effective (depending on your business, of course) with a sweater-and-skirt ensemble. Low-heeled shoes even with an added bow or flower can look wonderful with pants or even with the unmatched suit.

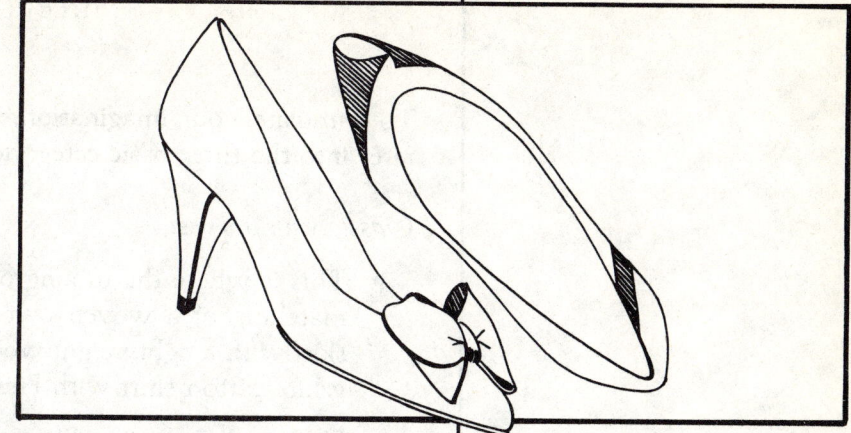

Strappy shoes are never appropriate, but you can wear slingbacks or open-toes. Just don't wear toenail polish. (Let them focus on your head, not your feet.) Always have on hand two pairs of neutral color, comfortable, medium-heeled shoes. (Stack heels have a tendency to look overly casual.) Why not buy one pair with bows or geometric color designs to add femininity and interest to your overall impression?

Now is the chance to bring in faux lizard pumps, racy colors, offbeat details, and clip-ons for shoes. Match hose with shoes to create a long, color-coordinated line which adds to an overall, pulled-together effect. On the other hand, with flat shoes, natural-toned hose is classic.

JEWELRY: Go to glorious excess in shapes, sizes, and colors, mixing beads and chains, gold with pearls, and remember to include hair combs or pouffs in highlighting colors. Earrings play an especially important part with less dressy separates, making them a touch more formal without overdoing. Bracelets, too, go well with separates, especially pants. Colored crystal beads are wonderful with unmatched suits. Chokers or beads that hang in long strands add decoration to tailored clothes and provide a very feminine touch. Classic gold or silver earrings, a good no-nonsense watch, and geometric pins make suitable choices for jackets, vests, and unmatched suits.

SCARVES: There are many ways to wear scarves (see Chapter 5, page 91); all of them have the effect of softening and feminizing the rest of your apparel. Go for quality scarves, but let your tastes roam from hunting scenes to floral prints. Frame your face with a paisley or dotted scarf wrapped around your neck.

"One of my summer outfits is a white blazer with a black linen skirt, a crisp white blouse, wide black belt, pale-white hose, and gold jewelry."

Personnel Director

Three Types

To stimulate your imagination, here's a breakdown of separates into the three basic categories.

Classic with a Twist

- This is where the mixing of textures shows, as in the matching of a woven rayon black-on-black patterned skirt with a lightweight wool pindot jacket and a crisp, white cotton shirt with French cuffs.

- Update that denim skirt with a black blazer, a black bowler with a blue floppy silk flower pin, and a blue paisley scarf with a sailor tie.

- A below-the-hips black blazer should have silver buttons to set it off. Team it with a wide fichet-collared white crisp cotton blouse, a slim chartreuse and black houndstooth skirt, and black hose.

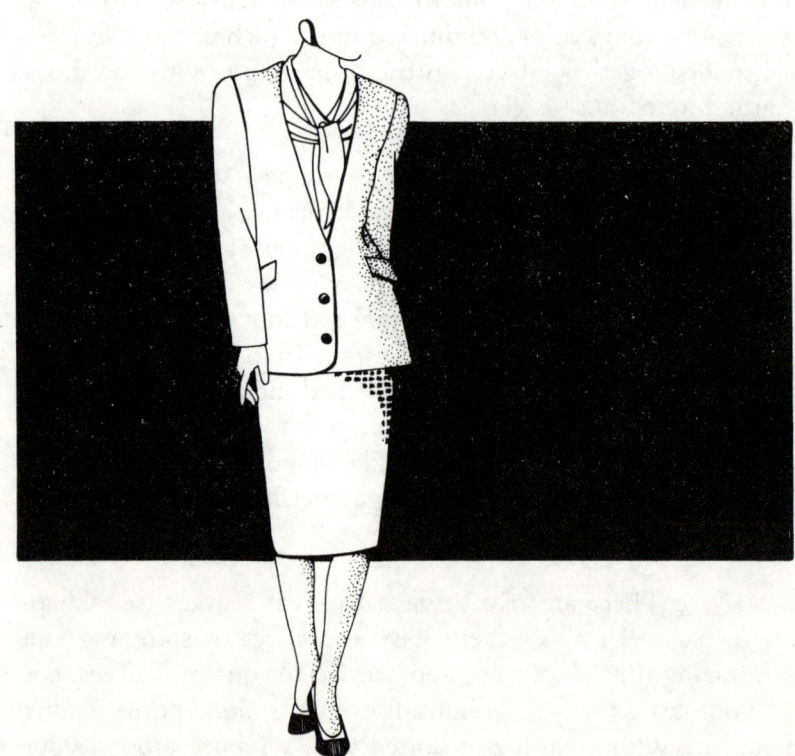

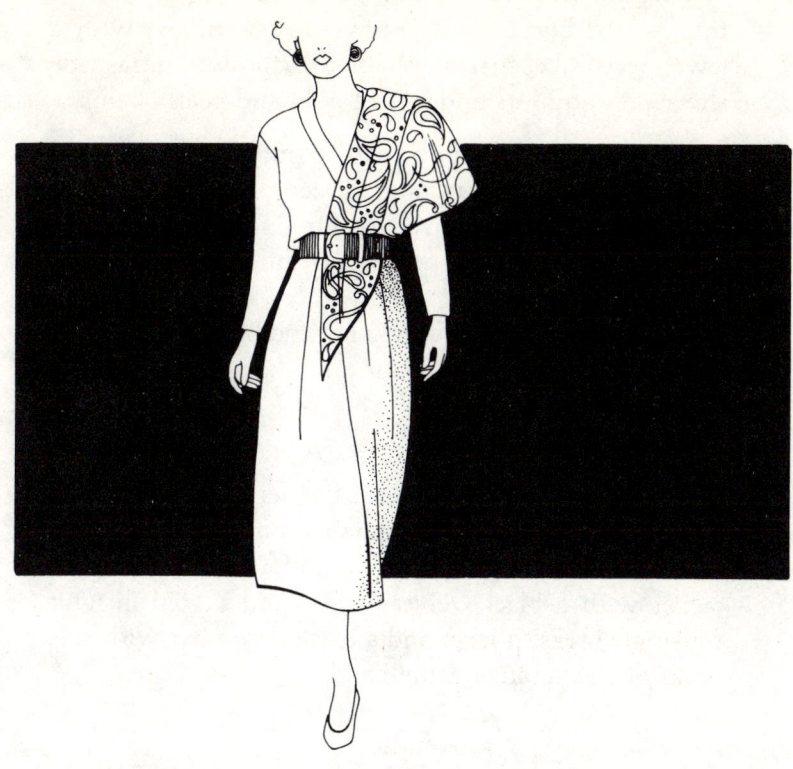

- A black, white, and red plaid short-cropped wool jacket can go nicely with a red silk notched-collar blouse and a short, slim black gabardine skirt.

- A muted sandstone-striped wool/rayon/silk jacket works with a softly pleated wool/crepe skirt, a wide brown belt, and, believe it or not, a purple poly/silk blouse with a self scarf.

- A white peplum jacket with gathers on either side, and black buttons will instantly come alive with amethyst earrings and gloves.

- Orange checks in a bolero jacket goes well with muted earth-orange pants in a smaller check. A rust blouse with a turned-up collar and bow earrings with a jade teardrop make this a classic.

- An extra-full jersey wool blouse with a shawl collar tucked into a wide black belt over a solid-colored skirt is finished off nicely with a large paisley shawl.

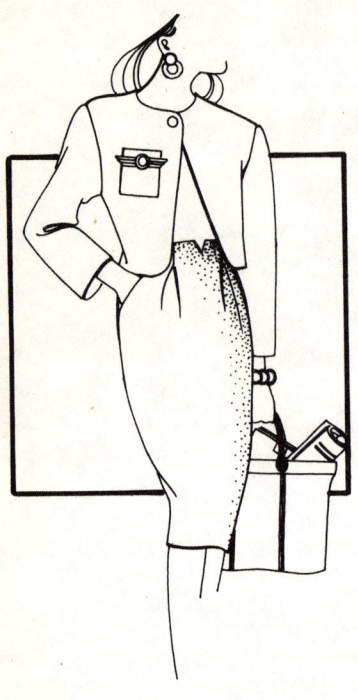

- A neat brown-and-white wool plaid long-line jacket may sound boring, but not when it is mixed with a jewel-neck silk charmeuse blouse, brown ultrasuede slim skirt, and lots and lots of gold and pearl chains.

- A conventional high-powered herringbone beige wool jacket still hanging around in your closet? Match it with a dark-brown wool crepe slim-line skirt and a huge herringbone scarf wrapped round and round.

- Wear a deep-red jacket with a red and black plaid dirndl. Add a wide black belt. Wear a red hat.

Avant-Garde

- A high-rise black rayon/wool flannel skirt worn with a Windsor-collared white pima cotton shirt, and a double row of black buttons, will set off a red short-cropped jacket with a black velvet collar. Add a gold insignia on single breast pocket and a black derby hat with two rows of gold coins on the band.

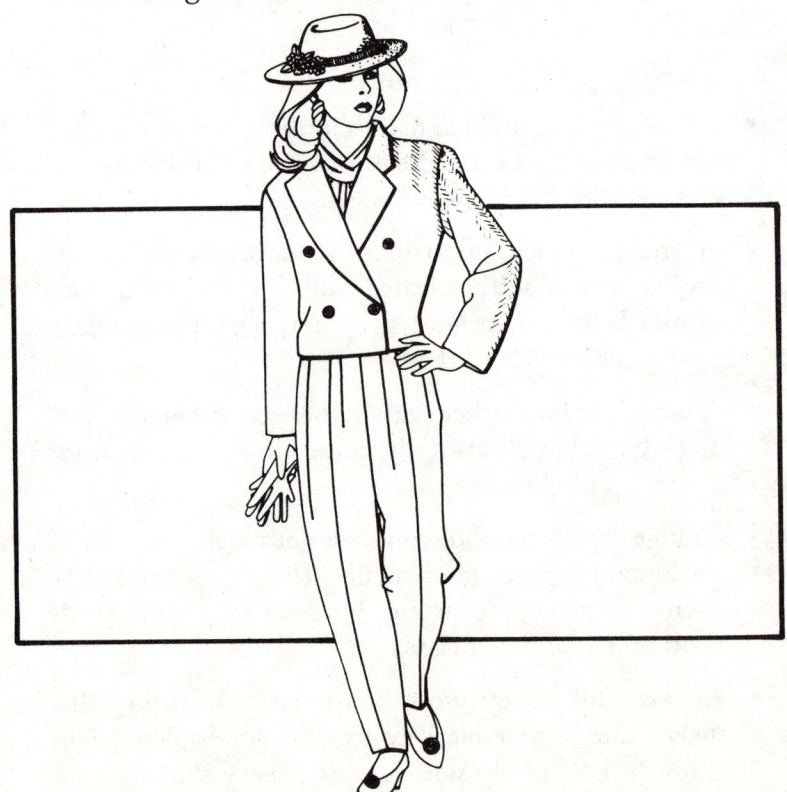

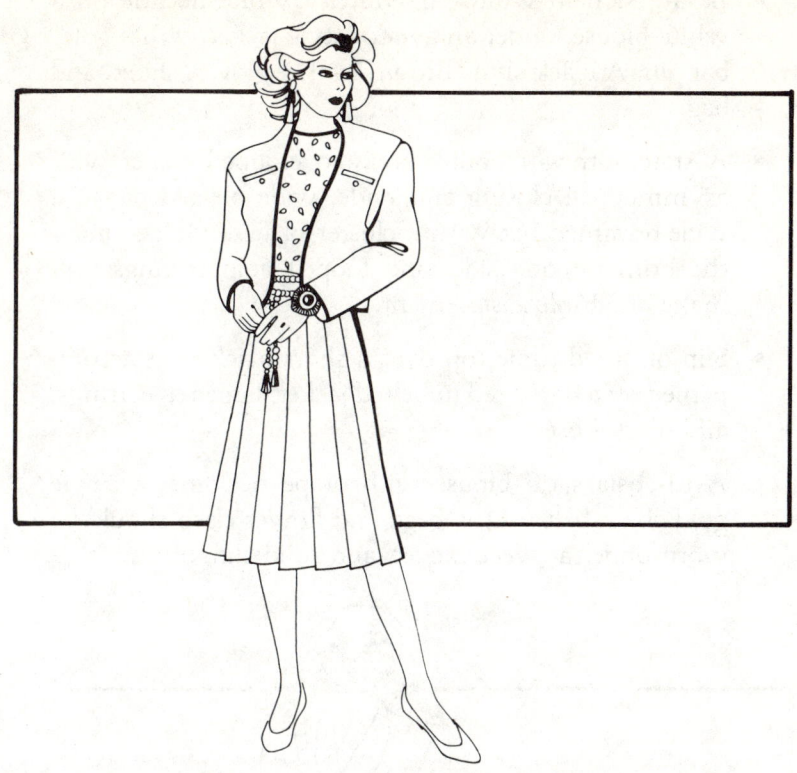

- Blues on blues. A venetian-layered blue skirt works with a wide black leather belt with a gold buckle and gold chains that loop it into place, and with a blue poly/silk blouse, with a deep, almost midnight-blue flower at the throat and a deep-blue jacket in soft lines.

- Try no collar on either a single-buttoned jacket with wide shoulders or a blouse underneath which should be the same color, and an aviator's pin on the breast pocket. Add a contrasting colored skirt.

- Purple jewelry will set off a side-buttoned black blouse that can be worn outside as a light jacket over a purple and black houndstooth sarong-style skirt. Carry a purple handbag in suede.

- If your black-and-white patterned jacket is made of a soft, drapey fabric such as woven rayon, it can go over a black-patterned skirt with a wide black belt tucking in the jacket at the waist. Under it, wear a gray jersey blouse with a self tie.

- Be a vision in white on white: a white necktie on a white blouse, under an aviator-style jacket with a gold-bar pin. A black skirt. Brown leather gloves, shoes, and bag.

- A state-of-the-art double-breasted cropped blazer with asymmetrical closing and wide, wide pleated pants, a wide-brimmed hat with a cluster of fake violets under the brim on one side, and looped gold earrings will make an absolute statement.

- Slip on a red tunic top over a short black skirt accompanied by a flared red unbelted jacket, large red earrings, and black hose.

- A fuschsia satin blouse with drape neckline, a single gold chain belt with a bead and flower clasp should be worn under a tweed jacket, and solid slim-line skirt.

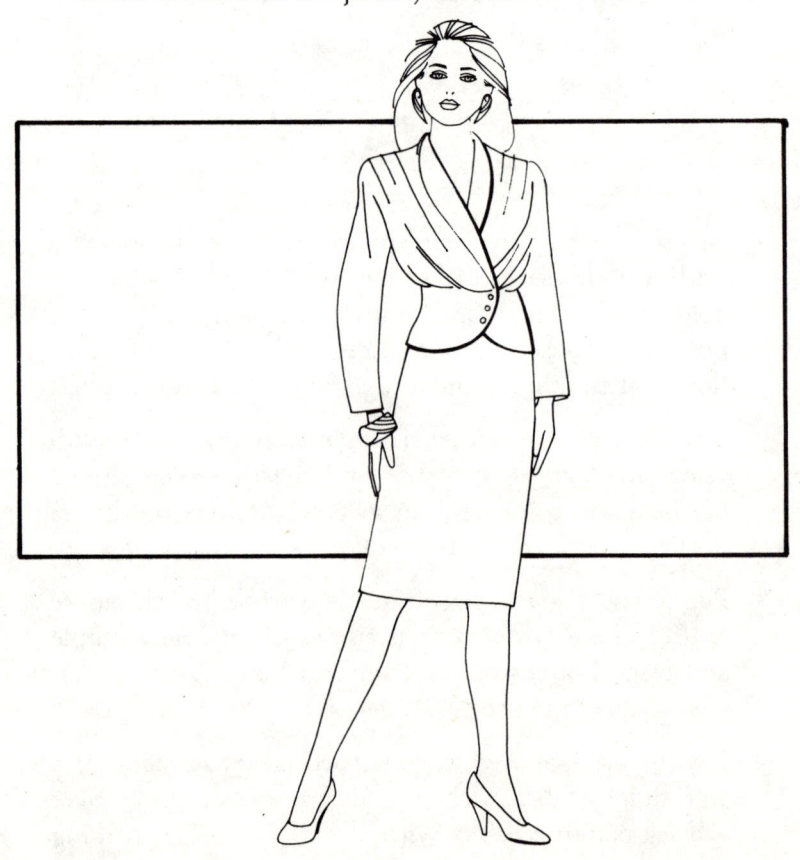

- Choose a chain belt with a front row of beads and tassels and a bracelet with a single gold sunburst and a center faux gem. Team these with a knife-pleat skirt, a wool/crepe soft-line buttonless jacket.

- Combine a pale-beige paisley skirt with a short-cropped black bolero, beige silk self-tie blouse bowed, and a newsboy cap.

- A conventional paisley in a long-line silk charmeuse jacket is made unconventional by teaming it with a matching shawl-collared blouse, a bright-red belt, and a navy wool slim-line skirt with a back slit.

- Add an avant-garde touch to that black–and–white houndstooth cropped jacket with a white silk poppy pin with a black center on one side of the jacket, and in the breast pocket, a saucy black-and-white polka-dot silk pouchette.

- A houndstooth jacket upon houndstooth pants, a black derby hat and a dash of red leather in gloves and pumps will make a strong, tasteful statement.

- A many-ruffled blouse with ruffles down each sleeve and a high collar can be teamed with a chain belt. This will have to be worn with a dramatic wool shawl in stripes or paisley, and a solid-toned soft-line pleated pants.

- A silk jersey blouse which wraps round and round into a modified peplum waist can act as a jacket over a slim skirt in bold plaid. Clunky gold jewelry will be needed with this outfit to set it off.

- Pair a cream wool flannel wide-lapeled long-line jacket with a cream jersey high-neck wrap blouse, a short lightweight silk camel skirt with a wide black belt, and a black flower shoe clip or antique brooch.

- Take a basic red skirt, wear it with a red-and-black print blouse, add a full red-and-black loose-style wool jersey jacket in a different print, and a black belt for a dynamite look.

Exotic

- Chartreuse is an exotic color in itself. When it shows up in a silk blouse with a drawstring that gathers at the waistline and ties in a bow, over a slim black skirt, accompanied by an oversize chartreuse houndstooth loose-fitting jacket, you have a double-dare exotic look.

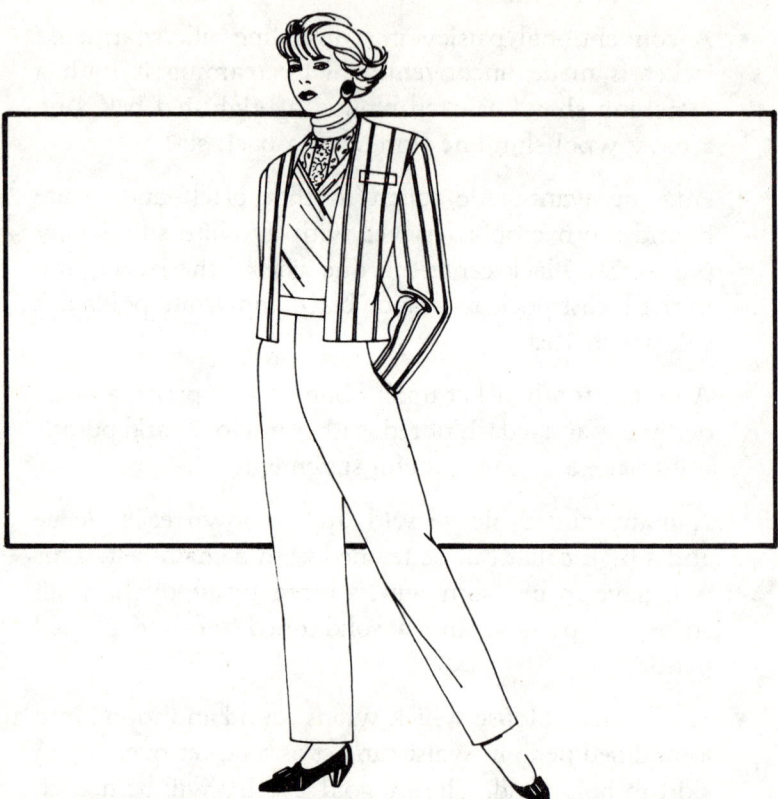

- Try a pink jacket over a pink-and-black flowered shirt, tucked into a black tiny-checked skirt.

- Slip on a paisley fitted jacket with dripping black/gold earrings.

- Take a deep-blue wool/crepe dirndl and pair it with a black short-cropped jacket and top with a blue/black/gold wool challis paisley stole. Add a faux wildberry bracelet and earrings.

- Wear all paisley: jacket, skirt, and roll-brimmed hat. Carry an art-deco plastic bag.

- Button up a high high-collared blouse with embroidery and lace inset in a deep V-yoke paired with a black wide-legged jumpsuit, and a black-and-white striped jacket.

- Ruffles to your ears in a full-collared blouse, and wide ruffles showing below jacket cuffs can be lovely if it is matched with an unsuspecting herringbone jacket and slim-line skirt. Balance is key here.

- Don't know what to wear with a green jacket? It goes very well with a black blouse and skirt, of course, black gloves, black hose and shoes, and a black with a green/purple fluffy flower pin.

- For utter elegance try an ultrasuede vest and jacket with a gray flannel skirt, and three neck scarves wound together and tied in a bow.

- Team a navy bankers'-striped skirt with a navy double-breasted jacket, and a wide-collared white-and-navy striped blouse. Wear it with red Bakelite beads and red shoes.

- An ivory silk shirt? Just add a nip-and-tuck black satin vest, a slim-line charcoal skirt, and a garnet/amethyst necklace of loops and loops. Over that slip a long-line wool and rayon tweed wide-checked jacket with red flecks.

- Fasten a pearl pin on a huge lacy neck scarf worn over a glen plaid jacket, solid-toned dirndl, and orange beads.

- Enjoy polka dots in a blouse hidden away, but not quite, under a striped jacket and a one-toned skirt. Wear a striped ponytail scarf.

- Team red, yellow, and black for a dashing, futuristic effect.

- Add a pink belt with a large silver ornate buckle to an otherwise staid black-and-white ensemble.

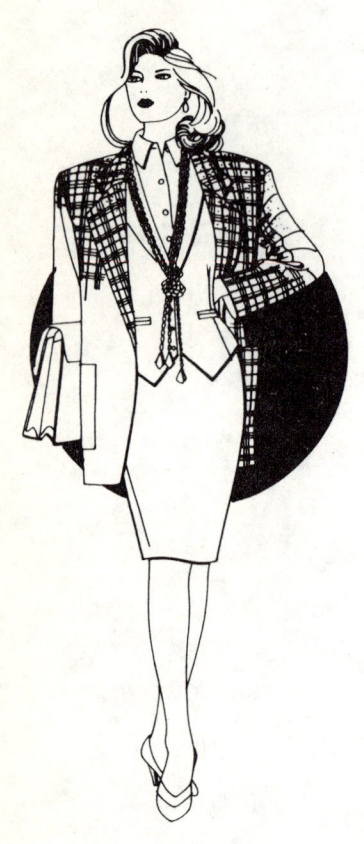

- Instead of conservative pearl earrings with a black slim skirt and short houndstooth jacket, wear funky earrings and a shawl wrapped around the waist to give the skirt high definition.

- A teal-blue double-breasted short-cropped blazer will instantly exoticize and update a plain black blouse and skirt, especially if you wear an antique gold pendant.

- An all-red jacket, all-red skirt, and underneath? Teal-blue blouse, blue hat and, no, not blue, but *red* shoes.

Dos and Don'ts

Do

Add accent color with a pin, a scarf, a belt, or a bag or shoes.

Strive for a strong statement BUT simplicity in accessorizing.

Become bolder with colors.

Find someone to give you feedback as to what works with your figure in terms of color, fit, and style.

Break color rules, including anything that limits you to a particular "season."

Shop small boutiques in addition to large department stores. Here you will be more likely to find individualistic looks that suit you better, and also receive more guidance.

Maximize your figure strong points; minimize your weak points. If you have good legs, don't be afraid to wear a skirt grazing the top of the knee.

Take a chance with patterns that you wouldn't ordinarily think would go together. Find some common thread of color or theme and see if it works or clashes.

Don't

Wear hose darker than your skirt.

Wear shoes that have no connection with any other part of your outfit.

Go above the knee with a hemline, unless your legs are terrific and the length allows only a modest glimpse.

Patronize the little-girl look.

Be afraid to put plaids with dots or stripes.

Hold back from separates thinking they are too casual. Separates expand a wardrobe and offer choices you don't otherwise have. Instead use accessories to help add formality.

Avoid sweaters. When chosen carefully, an expensive sweater that fits in an eased fashion can convey an elegant femininity that is hard to match.

Skimp on shoes, bags, or umbrellas. They, too, must spell out quality and taste.

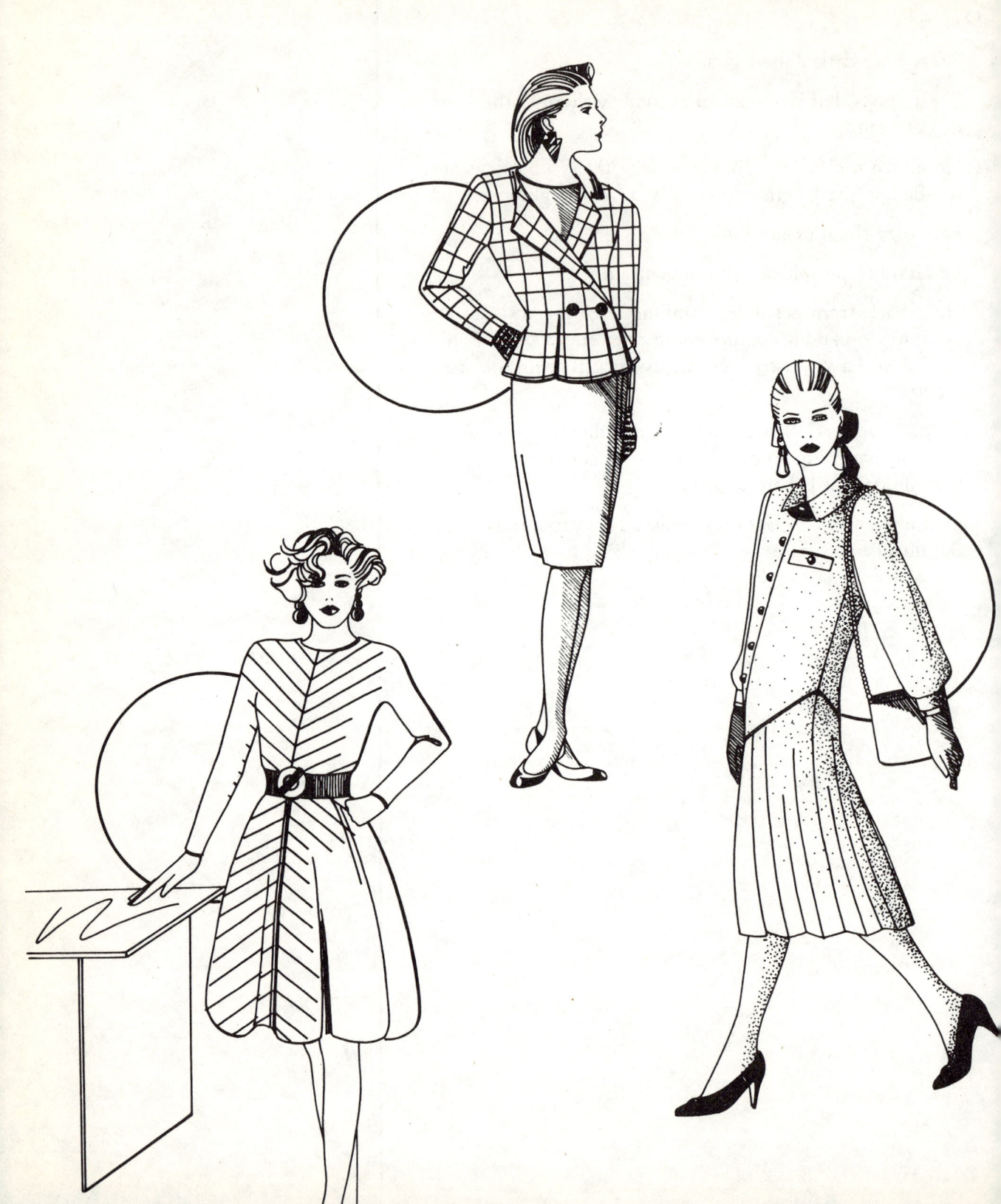

Dresses That Work

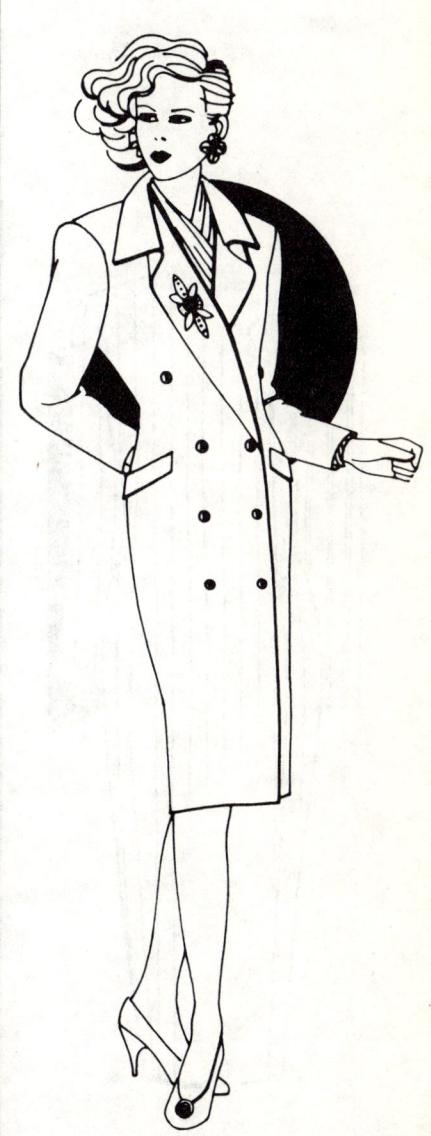

Dresses are refreshingly easy to wear and deliciously feminine. As women first began surging into executive positions, we disregarded dresses as being too feminine for the office. And they were. For two reasons. The styles did not reflect serious business intent, and the workplace was not prepared to view *any* dress as truly appropriate for high-level positions.

This is no longer true. The new freedom to look feminine and professional at the same time is a sweep that includes dresses, and they are appearing in power scenes. TV anchorwomen wear them; congresswomen wear them; vice presidents are wearing them. Manufacturers have been slow to respond, and seem to have trouble designing with the office in mind, but it *is* happening. More and more dresses are available in styles and colors that are appropriate for the office and offer greater versatility for our career-fashion closet.

How to Handle Dresses

The classic look is one of simplicity of line, quality of fabric, and elegant details. Professional dresses usually have long

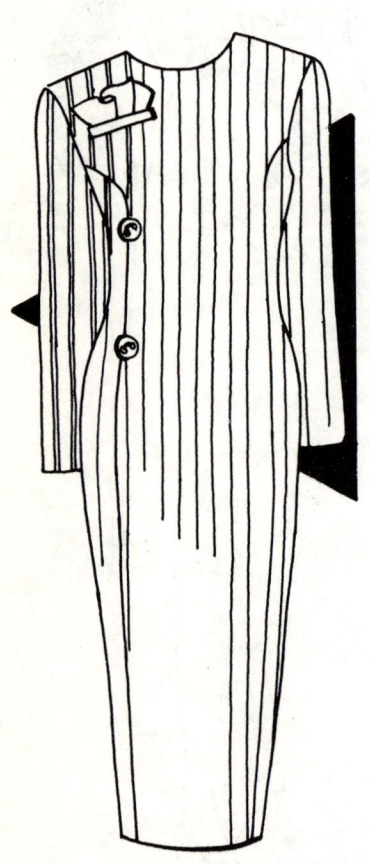

sleeves and either a slim-line skirt or a softly gathered one. The classic *coatdress* and the *shirtwaist* are style staples. The *chemise*, which has no waistline and is lately quite short, comes and goes in fashion cycles. Chemises are a particular style and therefore have a shorter fashion life. They provide a pleasant change of pace. *Wrap dresses* are highly feminine yet not overtly sexy, and so they, too, fit into a professional routine. All of these styles, depending on cut and fabric, are generally appropriate for a woman executive, depending on the professional field.

CHEMISES: The *chemise,* which falls from neckline to hem with barely a nip-in to indicate a waist, presents a sleek silhouette. A single button at the top of a cream poly/wool or even poly/crepe chemise makes for a dress simple enough to look businesslike, elegant enough to wear to the office and to dinner afterward. In poly/crepe it will be machine washable, too. One place where pinstripes continue to work is a lightweight wool chemise with perhaps two large buttons at the side of the bodice and a slash of a breast pocket just right for a bright pouchette. The only problem with a chemise is that it does not respond well to a jacket, and women executives still like to be able to wear a jacket with their dresses, although this is not de rigueur any more. A loose, unstructured jacket could possibly work with this silhouette. If you're shopping for chemises, take your jacket along so that it can be tried with the dress.

COATDRESSES: Belted, with large buttons, a *coatdress* is spectacularly classic in a European, old-world way. Its style is both businesslike *and* feminine. Coatdresses, like chemises, do not adapt well to a jacket. To avoid feeling "underdressed" without a jacket, add a wool challis stole or a huge silk-print scarf.

SHIRTWAISTS: Shirtwaists should be in a high-quality fabric to avoid looking overly casual. Cotton poplin, for instance, will not work at all. However, the same style in lightweight wool jersey, silk, or poly/silk, worn with a wide belt, conveys femininity as well as richness.

WRAP DRESSES: Wrap dresses are heavenly when it comes to comfort and are also thoroughly feminine. They come in florals, solids, small prints, and in a range of fabrics. Wool jersey fits this style beautifully.

Fit

With all clothes, fit is a crucial consideration. Style and color actually play secondary roles to the fit of clothing. Fit may be somewhat more relaxed with dresses, as compared to a suit with its need for precision tailoring. However, certain parameters must be followed if a dress is to enhance your feminine businesslike appearance.

Shoulders in a dress should hit your shoulder mark squarely. The back of the dress should not bulk up, the waist must hit at the waist unless it is a specifically high-waist or dropped-waist look (and a garment designed to fit the figureline is always better than one that is not supposed to fit and doesn't). Sleeves should end at the break of the wrist, and hems should fall at or just below the knee for a short dress, or mid-calf for a longer dress.

Coordinate these basic principles of fit with your own figure weaknesses and strengths. Apply them when buying a dress. They can also be beneficially applied to blouses and skirts.

Details

One of the reasons we like dresses so much is that they frequently come with flattering, soft details such as peplums, ruffles, tiered skirts, floral or geometric prints, self-sashes, or dropped waistlines. There is so much room for femininity and individuality in dresses, and designers seem to be just beginning to explore the potential of dresses suitable for business.

PLEATS: Today pleats show up in dresses, creating a feminin-

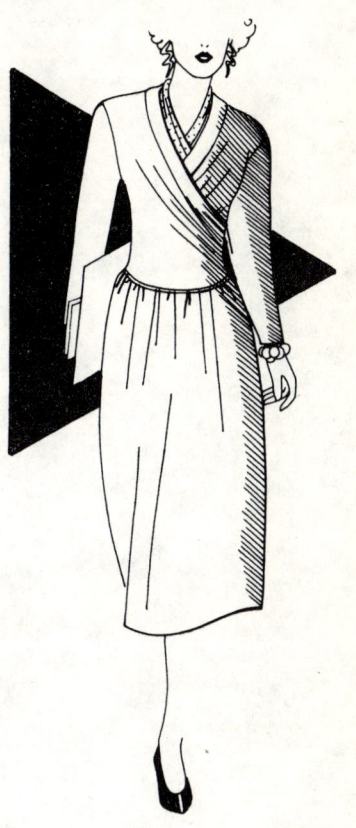

Elizabeth Dole started out as Duke University May Queen. Now she dresses with very little jewelry, going for tasteful soft-colored dresses with rope-chain necklaces.

87

ity of movement while maintaining a smooth silhouette and a formal quality.

SHOULDERS: Shoulders in dresses today are usually slightly rounded with small shoulder pads. If you have a favorite dress with yesterday's huge shoulder pads, simply replace them with smaller ones.

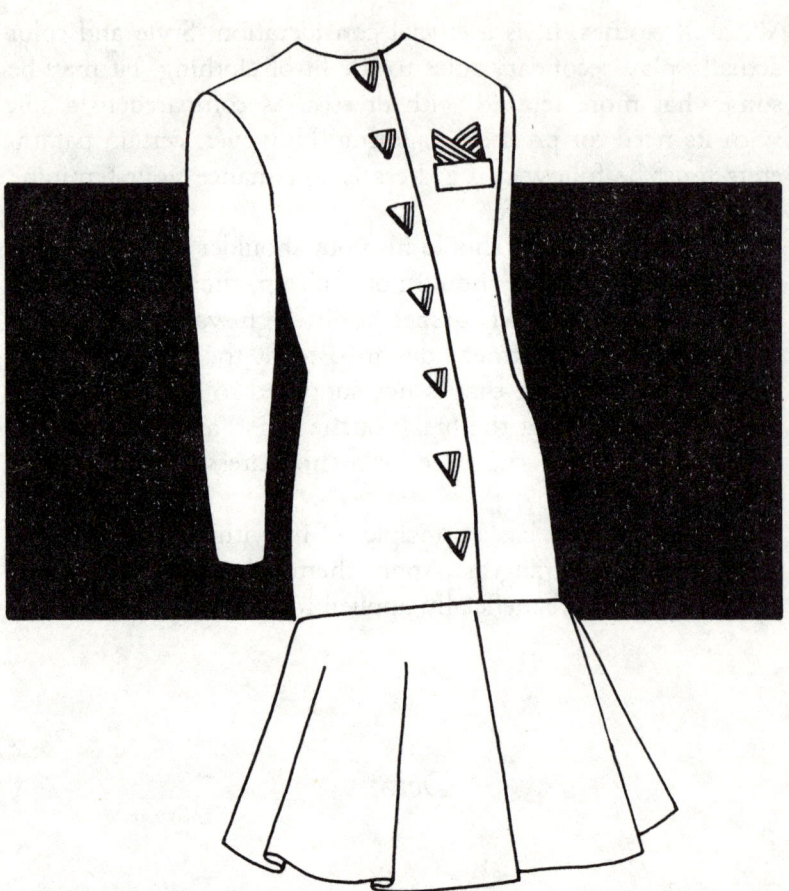

POCKETS: A dress may have pockets [usually hidden in a side seam], but they cannot be used in the same way as those on a suit jacket or skirt. They are not a place to put your hands or assorted pens and notes. Dress lines and the closer fit of a dress preclude bulky pockets. A full pocket interrupts the smooth draping of lighter, softer fabrics. The only thing you can keep in a dress pocket is a linen handkerchief or a business card. As for patch pockets, they are a detail that generally adds little. You can only use the pocket for a silk pouchette, and patch pockets tend to interfere with the effect of necklaces. Flap pockets look mannish and, again, cannot be utilized.

YOKES AND INSETS: Details such as V-*yoke* bodices, or inverted pleats in the back of the skirt do not make bold statements, but can add a graceful elegance. If the color and fabric of the dress are perfect for you, and if these details are handled subtly, they could be just the special touch that makes the dress unique. For yokes or insets to work depends on the quality involved.

BUTTONS: Obvious buttons are an accessory. They can either rescue a drab dress or interfere with a classic one. If you love the dress but hate the buttons, buy it and be creative with replacements. Or to update the look of a dress, simply replace the old buttons with better ones.

Having to compete with snaps, buttons, or flaps when you accessorize limits your ability to alter the effect of a dress. It is better to have a relatively plain dress for the optimum in versatility.

Fabrics

Lighter fabrics such as sheer wools, silks, poly/silk, a silky poly, and wool jersey are often used in dresses. Wool crepe is a dressy fabric but it is still suitable for career dressing in certain fields. A cascade-collared black coatdress in wool crepe can easily take you from the boardroom to client dinners in style.

Corduroy is a fabric that is too casual whether it shows up in a suit or a dress. Some firms ask their women executives not to wear it. Corduroy is best kept for country weekends.

Large plaids and the usual gamut of businesslike prints show up in dresses, along with floral designs, either bold or miniature. These days a silk flower pin often comes with a good dress. This can be used to hold a silk scarf in place, too.

"*Although most of my attire consists of suits, I have been wearing more dresses, especially in summer. In mix-and-match prints, too. I never would have thought of doing that before, but it's fun.*"
Bank Loan Officer

Colors

Color is an indulgence that dresses allow. Purples, reds, roses, and patterns in black/red, beige/black all show up in dress/jacket ensembles. A great deal of black and white abounds as a classic combination. Yet with all this, one of the best dress investments you can make is still the basic black. Team that with a black-and-white striped jacket, black hose, and black power pumps and you have a very chic new power look.

Pastels, including cream, yellow, and beige, although a touchy choice when it comes to businesswear, are fine if you live in the West or South. In summertime, they are generally more acceptable in offices everywhere. Little-girl shades such as baby pink and baby blue, should be avoided no matter where you live and work.

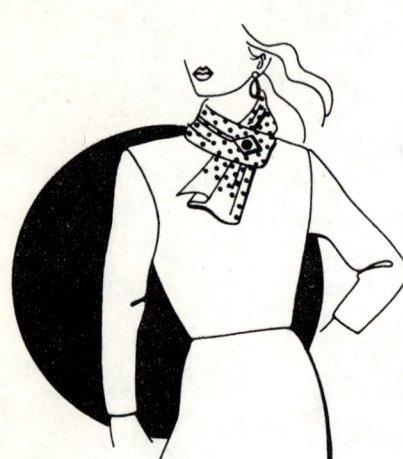

Jane Pauley favors patterned dresses, often in yellows, and accompanies them with gold earrings and a tailored hair bow on her sleek ponytail.

Accessories

NOTE: Each accessory changes the look. The wrong accessory can ruin the entire outfit. Beyond a certain point, too, adding accessories can detract from the success of your overall look.

SCARVES: Scarves add color, texture, and flair. Scarves work best with simple outfits. Don't do too much to accessorize them, perhaps add only gold earrings or a few gold chains. The outfit and the scarf may look special by themselves but together are all wrong. This is a matter of experimenting in front of a mirror.

You should own at least one large scarf, about 45″ x 45″, that you can throw around your shoulders as a shawl, or wrap around your waist; also a small scarf for the pocket [pouchettes], and a long narrow one to tie into a neck bow or use as a sash. Colors should complement your complexion as well as the basic tones in your wardrobe.

Go for wide scarves, the best you can buy. Oblongs make a good bow, close to the neck or loose, either under a collar or

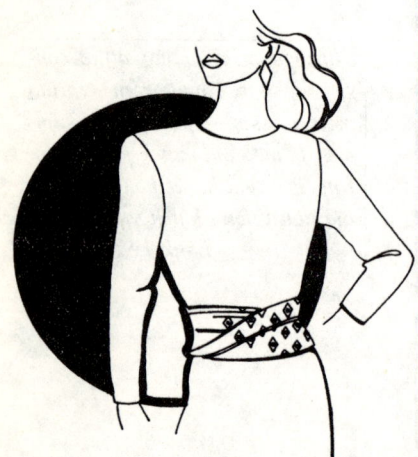

over a jewel neckline. Use also as a cummerbund, ascot, or muffler under coats.

Tie a scarf to one side of the neck, pin over one shoulder or fold triangularly like a sash from shoulder to waist and belt into place. This works well with jackets or knit dresses.

Wear bright scarves with dark winter colors, even two to three at once, too, in new, jewel tones.

Ways to tie scarves: Bow at the neck in the shape of a flower. Fold into a band and stick into a pocket. Tie scarves sailor style or man-tie style, or wrap twice around the neck, make one end into a bow puff, the other end can hang down under this. Fold in half (a long, oblong scarf) for a self loop. Also wear with the point in front.

Wear a large scarf around the neck, tied to one side or clipped with a pin at the waist (depending on your waistline).

Pouchettes are tiny scarves in bright colors that can instantly update a look in bright blue, pink, or green, and go into a pocket just like a handkerchief. They are especially wonderful on a simple white or black dress.

Scarves in stripes, polka dots, with horses (ranchy) or dogs

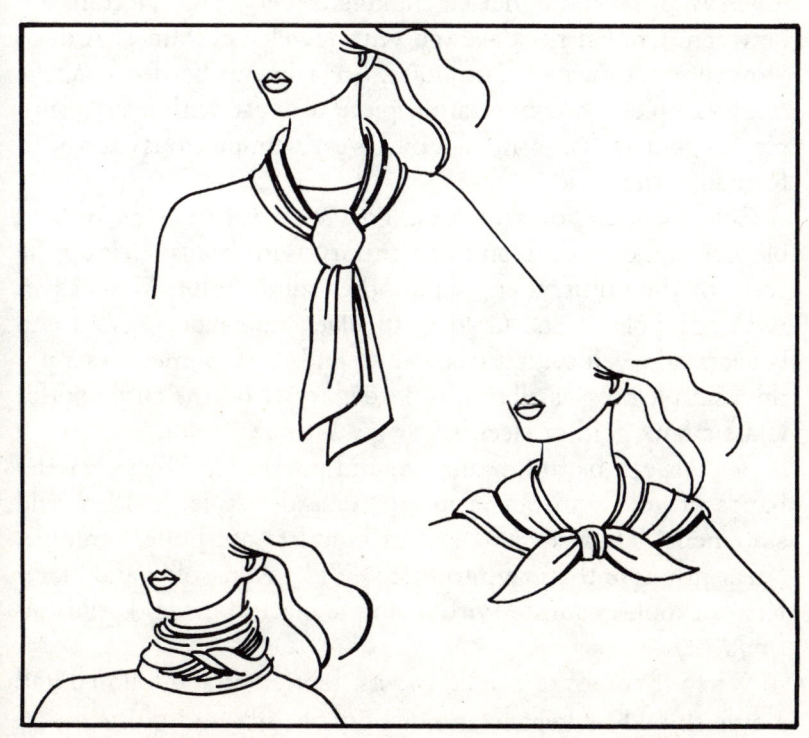

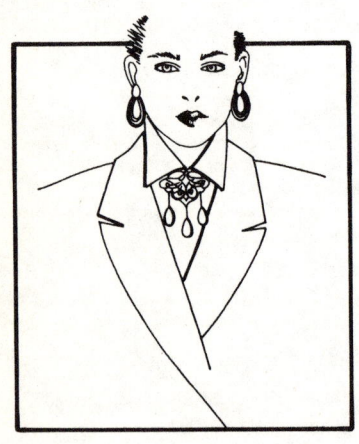

are chic. Black-and-white stripes go well with bright red jewelry, but black-and-white polka dots do not go well with pearls.

JEWELRY: The more elaborate the jewelry, the more simple the outfit should be. If the outfit is busy, use less jewelry or none at all. Faux or costume jewelry can look very chic. Heavy gold is best. You want jewelry to be fairly large while at the same time avoid appearing weighted down. The trick is not to wear too much jewelry in the business world, but to select one or two items, such as a necklace (or several, if they are pearls and chains) and earrings, and avoid overdoing with rings, bracelets, and pins.

People notice *earrings* in particular. They are easy to buy and can instantly make you feel more pulled together. They also go with most things which eliminates at least one worry about mixing and matching. The point to keep in mind with all jewelry is appropriateness and tastefulness. Sometimes a small face can carry large earrings. It depends on how they frame your face. Two pairs of earrings is generally enough to cover all business fashion requirements.

Necklaces should either be chokers or very long. Nothing in-between. Choker necklaces go with jewelry necklines. A dyed Howelite necklace, in turquoise, on a heavy beaded chain is one example of a conversation piece to wear with a very simple, elegant dress. With a knit, wear semiprecious stones to formalize the look.

Colorful long rows of *beads* go well with vests as well as blouses and dresses. Don't be contrary with beads. Pick up the color of the outfit, then add another subtle color. Wear silver with red polka dots. Gold with black polka dots. Gold and black work well with a tropically vivid scarf. Sometimes a pin on a simple dress is all that is needed to set off the entire outfit. Classic faux gold or sleek silver go with any color.

Bracelets can be fun, feminine, and interesting. Wide bracelet bands of gold with jewel inserts, crusader style, make a bold statement. Thin silver Mexican bracelets are quite feminine. Wear no more than two to three. Wide plain gold band bracelets can look exquisite with a simple black dress and gold earrings.

When it comes to *hair accessories,* fabric ties and tailored hair bows should be kept in mind. Bows in silk and grosgrain are suitable for office wear. Velvet is not. Stripes and polka dots can sometimes be slipped into an executive style, too, depending on your career field.

BELTS: To make any dress sleeker, add a wide belt, lightly tinted hose (never wear hose darker than your skirt or shoes), chains, beads, or silk scarf.

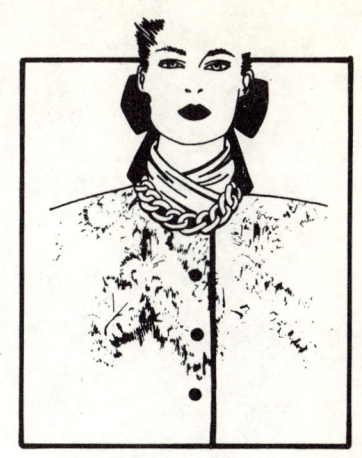

Three Types

Classic with a Twist

- A black dress can go so many ways. Choose one with a dropped waist in a wool double knit, rounded shoul-

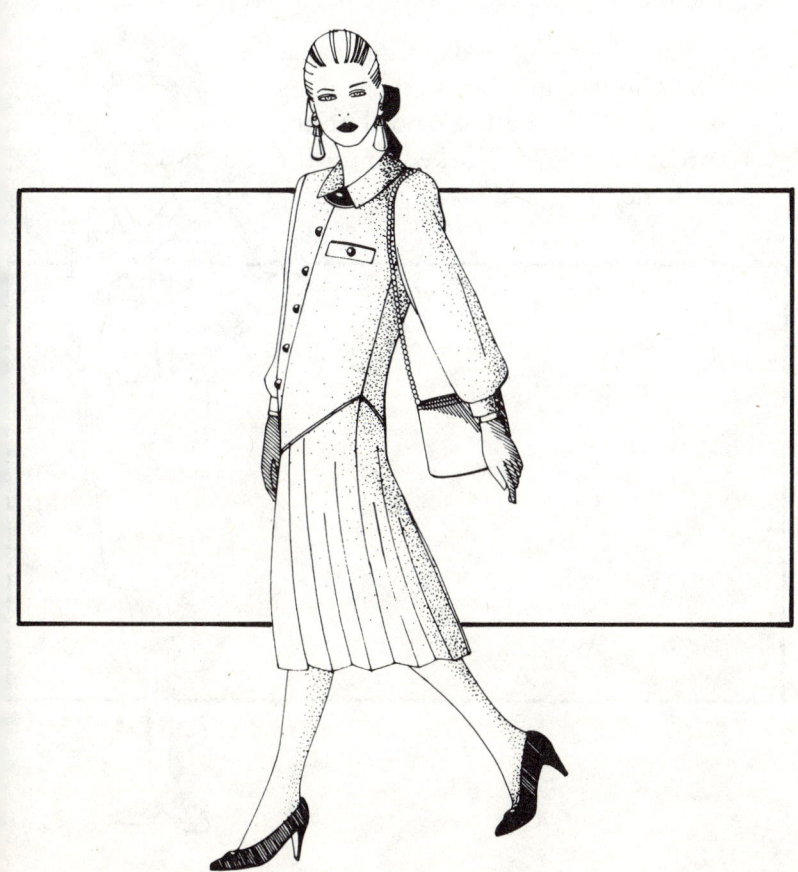

der pads, and a deep stitched V-yoke. With it wear nothing but huge gold earrings, black suede pumps, black leather gloves, and carry a black bag. The effect will be stunning. Or do the same with a black chemise in silk crepe which needs no belt.

- Take the black silk crepe chemise and pair it with a chartreuse bag.

- A gray flannel chemise to the knee top, worn with a glen plaid or a bright-red wool long-line jacket can be very elegant. Wrap a scarf round and round at the neck.

- With a black-and-white striped, full-sleeved, notch-collared wrap dress, add a huge floppy flower-shaped pin and gold earrings.

- To a classic pin-striped blue wool chemise with two large side buttons, add a navy printed pocket scarf in the breast pocket and wear a plain navy hat.

- A gold chain belt updates the classic black dress with slim sleeves, along with a white scarf wrapped at the throat, the ends tucked into the neckline, plus gold/black earrings.

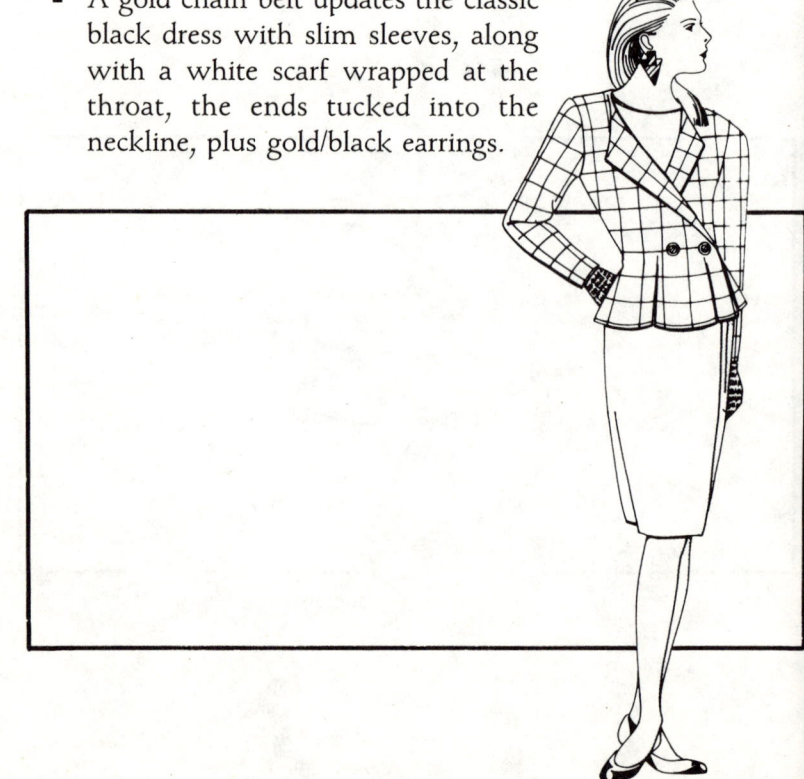

- A black-checked dress? Wear with a matching black-checked jacket, black hose and black leather gloves, and red patent leather pumps with a black bow.

- A classic coatdress, double-breasted, in purple! All that needs is large, geometric gold earrings with a purple stone setting.

- Another way to update the black dress: Wear a gold single-breasted blazer, black hose, black gloves, and a clunky gold necklace and earrings.

- Wear a black-and-white striped long-line blazer with a black dress and huge red earrings.

Avant-Garde

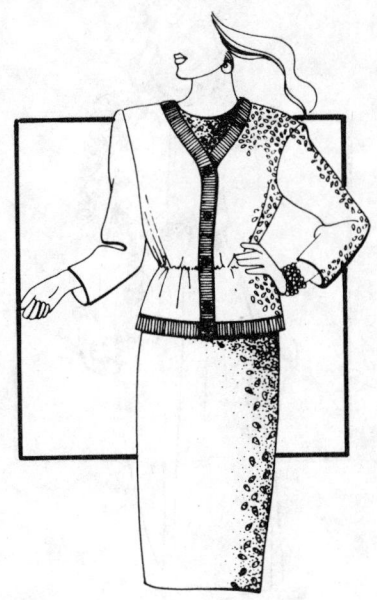

- Wear a short-cropped black wool double-breasted jacket with a standup collar, over a black silk dress. Add silver/black earrings.

- To set off that red wool dress, wear it with a red plaid, double-breasted peplum jacket, black-and-red gloves, black hose, and black shoes with a red geometric pattern.

- Take a plain gray wool sheath and add a houndstooth peplum jacket in fuchsia, purple, or black. Wear gloves and a scarf in gray or black.

- A coat-style dress with a wide skirt in oversize plaid with a wide belt and gold earrings.

- A fitted chemise in a mottled two-toned pattern such as red/black with a floral-print silk scarf.

- A tent-wide chemise with narrow fitted arms in neon chartreuse.

- Belt an earth-toned plaid jacket over a gray flannel dress. Pick up the tones in earrings and wear a bold gold necklace and earrings.

- Add a black-and-cream patterned woven rayon jacket with a black-on-black patterned slim-skirted dress.

- A long long-line black-and-white checked jacket with

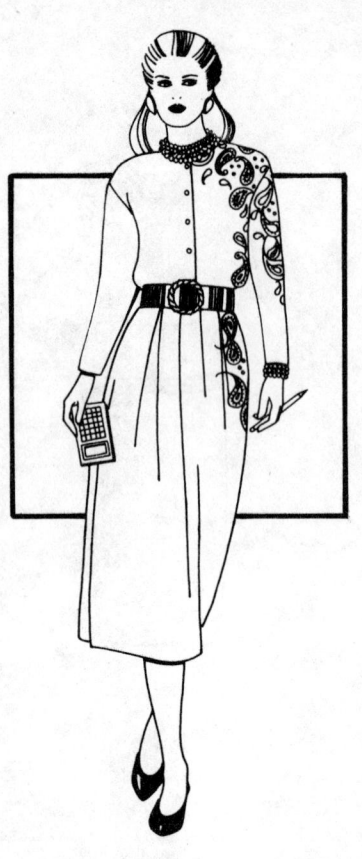

black buttons, and a black houndstooth shoulder stole, over a slim red or blue dress works beautifully. Add gold earrings with a setting that matches the dress.

- Try a red long-line jacket over a red slim dress, with red gloves and a gold/red pin. Add black-tone stockings and black pumps.

- A brown plaid dress with a purple pocket pouchette.

- A man-tailored blazer over a wrap dress with a cream silk aviator scarf and gold insignia pin.

Exotic

- Have your cake and eat it too with a two-piece challis dress in multi-colored paisley. A paisley-colored choker accentuates this look. Use an entirely different accent color in belt and gloves.

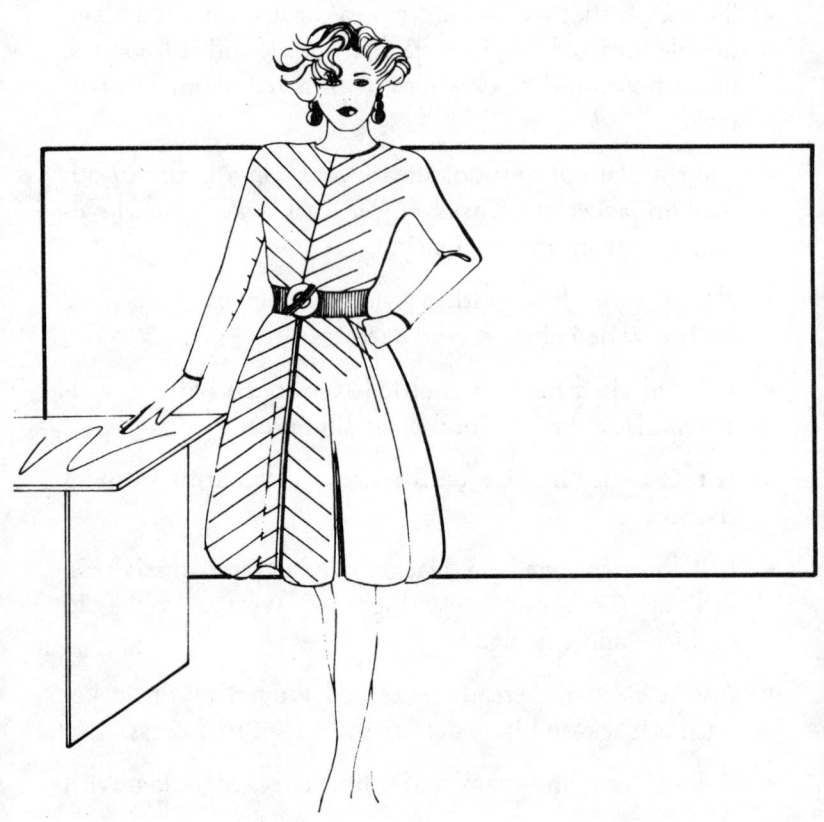

- Play against the obvious with a black soft-skirted dress with a wide brown leather belt, brown woven leather shoes, and a brown bag. Add black-and-gold earrings.

- Team a cream wool dress with a challis paisley jacket, and a lace handkerchief in the breast pocket.

- A black-and-white striped dress with a pouf-skirt, a three-inch belt with a giant circle clasp, and drop earrings.

- A jade-green wrap dress with a giant wrap shawl in green/gold/red in silk and gold jewelry.

- Wear a black-and-white polka-dot scarf ascot style with a gold clip over a black/gray thin-striped shirtdress with a black belt.

- A wool jersey can work as a wrap jacket over a multi-valanced skirted dress.

- Tie three scarves in complimentary color tones at the neck to liven up a camel-colored coatdress.

- A pindot chemise with kick pleats of polka dots and a huge polka-dot neck scarf in contrasting color. Two watches with different colored polka-dot bands are a bright chic addition.

- A subtly flowered dress combined with a glen plaid long-line jacket of the same colors. Butterfly pin with faux gems to underline the colors.

- Throw on a purple tweed jacket over a long, slim black dress.

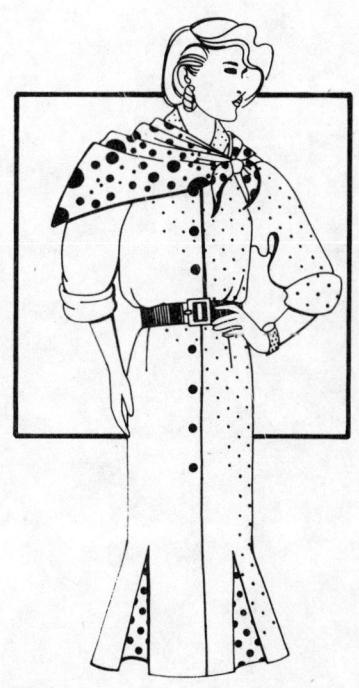

Dos and Don'ts

Do

Wear a lacy pocket handkerchief as a dress accessory.

Snip off a self neck bow from a dress and replace it with

a huge floppy silk bow in contrasting stripes or polka dots.

Wear a jacket with a short-sleeved dress in summer.

Replace flowery trim with piping for a more sleek appearance.

Accompany jewel necklines with jewelry—faux or real.

Consider buying dresses without collars. This provides the perfect background for great jewelry.

Wear blousons if your career allows. The style falls naturally in a loose, soft fabric such as rayon or rayon blend.

Choose side-wrap sarong-style dresses in formal fabrics only, such as soft wool. Otherwise, you'll look like you're on the road to Rio.

Cover a deep V-neckline with a soft scarf pinned into place.

Wear Chanel chains and pearls with an otherwise plain, though elegant, shirtwaist dress. (Don't roll up the sleeves.)

Buy shirtwaists and coat dresses in wool, wool jersey, or a good woven rayon.

Add a short-cropped or long-line jacket over a wrap dress.

Take off the self belt with a dress and use your own.

Don't

Wear dresses with yard-wide skirts, no matter how swingy they feel.

Buy flannel flowery shirtdresses touted as having "comfort and charm." Comfort and charm belong at home in the armchair.

Wear rhinestones to the office.

Wear little pins which look tiny and say nothing.

Wear dresses with white collars and self bows—too babyish and limiting.

Buy a dress with a knit collar or cuffs. The look is casual.

Wear sleeves that need pushing up in order for the dress to look good.

Wear a sweaterdress even in cashmere. This is bound to look clingy and sexy.

Wear a dress with a cutout neckline or back.

Select a dress in satin, velvet, or acetate which looks satin-ish.

Wear cotton knit dresses to work. In most professions they do not look suitably formal.

Allow an elasticized waistband to show. Cover it with a belt.

Wear a chemise in a jersey knit.

Wear a dress with a cutout back or a looped cutout neck, in any fabric but especially in a knit.

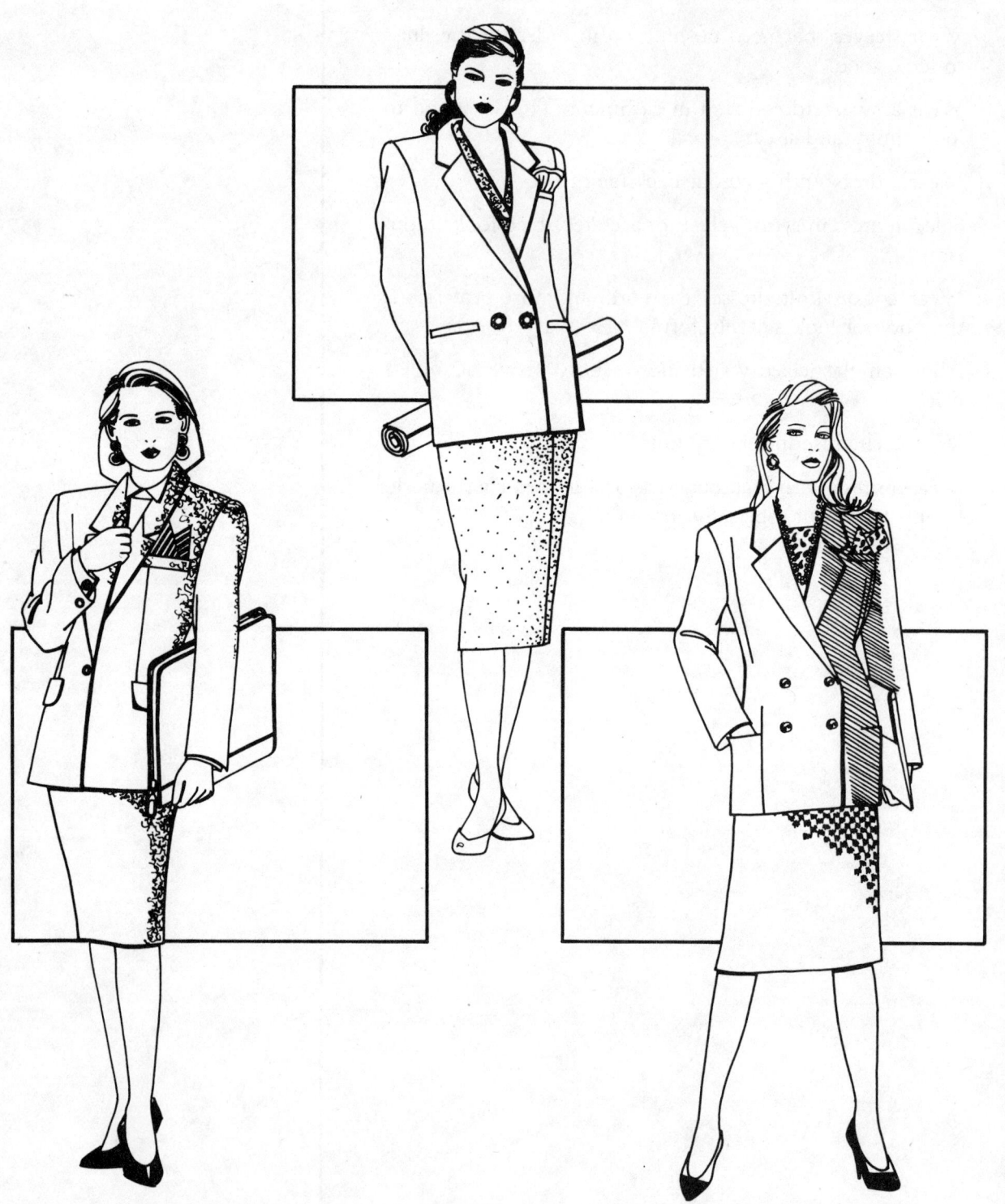

Right for the Occasion

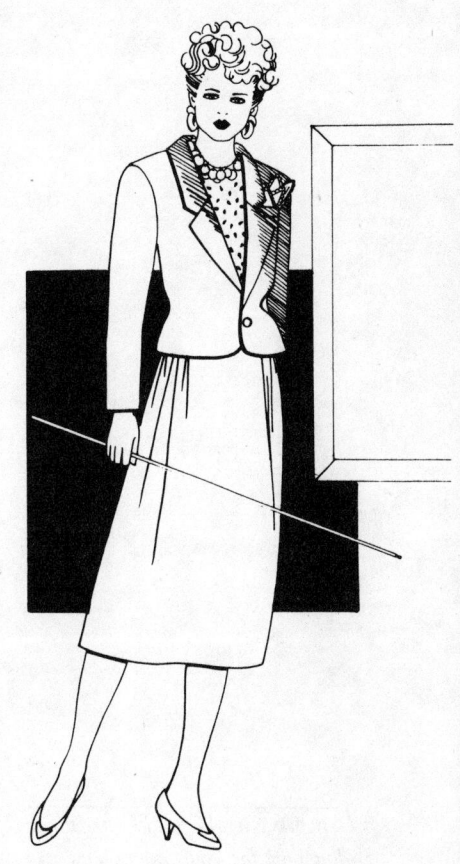

Every field has its own day-to-day standards. But it doesn't stop there. Different events within these fields, such as presentations, interviews, parties, picnics, dinners, all require a subtle and sometimes not-so-subtle changing of the rules within the general professional parameters. Of course, a certain commonality underlies these occasions, whatever the job, whatever the calling. Besides quality, neatness, comfort, and femininity without overt sensuality, what you want to convey always is responsibility, self-control, and an ability to play the game. All of this has to be considered when deciding what to wear to any business occasion, whatever the field. No matter what we choose to wear, the result must be creative but solid, in the spirit of the event, but controlled.

Presentations

Presentations mean walking or standing for a long period of time in front of a group of people. No matter the field, this calls for comfortable clothing, yet garments that will be eye-catching. Blouses should be long enough to stay tucked in so that you don't have to fidget and worry about them coming out at the waist. Skirts should not be uncomfortably tight, nor should they be shorter than the bottom of the knee. When you're in front of people, the best length is a conservative one. An elastic waistband on a skirt will let you breathe deeply which means you will be more relaxed. Anything that pinches your breathing should be avoided, as shallow breathing can easily promote tension. If you tend to perspire when nervous, wear a light fabric suit or dress, and avoid, for example, cashmere or flannel. In general, you want an outfit you can forget about.

To get and keep attention, choose something bright, or include brightly colored accessories so that people's minds don't wander too far away from you even if they aren't catching every word. However, if you wear something *too* bright or avant-garde, you may find that people concentrate too much on your appearance and not enough on your words.

Shoes must be ones you can tolerate standing and walking in for hours, perhaps all day. That means mid-heel, unless you have a high pain threshold, in soft Italian or woven leather. Everything about you will be scrutinized, so your tote, your eyeglass case, your handkerchief(s) must all be tip-top.

On the subject of handkerchiefs, you shouldn't still be carrying tissues when you could have Irish linen and lace with or without embroidery. Why miss a chance to make a subtly feminine statement?

Some Presentation Possibilities

- A cropped jacket and wool dirndl skirt with side buttons for extra interest.

- Cream jacket with jet skirt, jet necklace, and chartreuse suede pumps and bag.

- A red plaid dress with black beads and a wide black belt with black power pumps.

- A solid-black jacket with a paisley-print slim skirt and a paisley many-wrapped neck scarf, with lacy shirt cuffs showing at the sleeves.

Board Meetings

This is no time to get eclectic, right? Wrong. Not that you want to go wildly creative, but board meetings don't necessarily translate into tucked-up, buttoned-down submersion of your own fashion statement. Yes, you must go formal. This is the time to wear the quality wool worsted suit, the best classic suede pumps, the exquisite silk blouse; or in summer, the black linen suit with a fresh flower on the lapel and crystal beads. Generally speaking, it is not a good idea to wear a pants suit to a board meeting. You do *not* want to draw excessive attention to yourself in this situation. You do want to present a capable and competent impression, and this is true in any field, of course.

A dress with a jacket could be fine in these circumstances, for instance if it's a classic black dress with a wool-and-silk tweed jacket. Combine this with simple (though huge) gold earrings, and you have a winning combination.

Do not over-adorn. One accessory touch should do it. A belt is an excellent choice. It conveys a sense of style without a heavy hand. Gloves and hats make no sense in this situation, unless you are coming in from outside. Avoid hair bows and clips. (Cheap plastic hair clips should always be shunned—substituting instead faux tortoise-shell combs.)

Some Board Meeting Possibilities

- A windowpane plaid suit with a rose at the neck, a silk plaid shirt in tonally matching colors, sheer hose, and plain pumps.

- A paisley jacket with a solid-toned skirt and a paisley scarf, plain pumps, and gold jewelry.

- A patterned two-tone blouse with a red jacket, a houndstooth skirt, and a red paisley pocket pouchette.

- A wrap jacket in power pindots with a polka-dot blouse, a striped pocket square, or a lace pocket handkerchief.

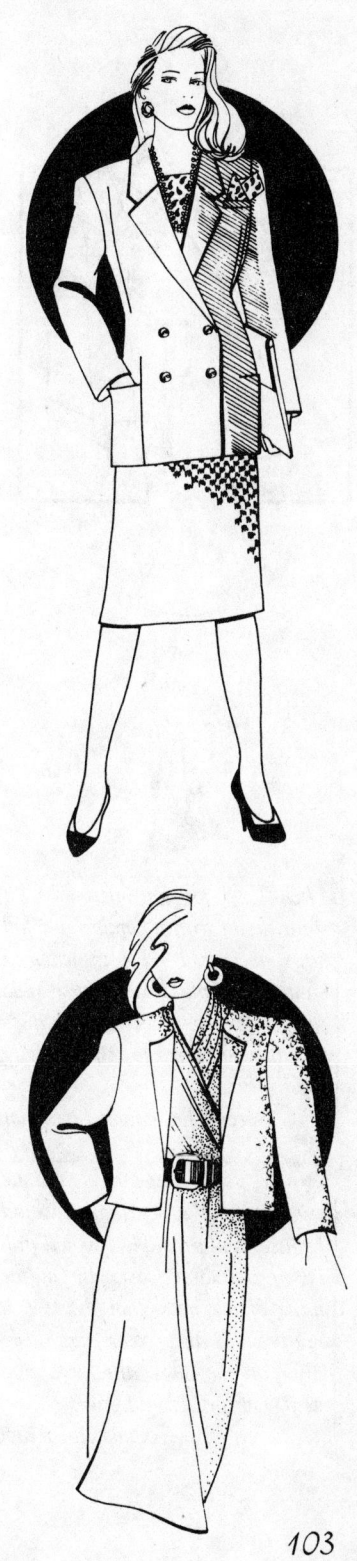

Interviews

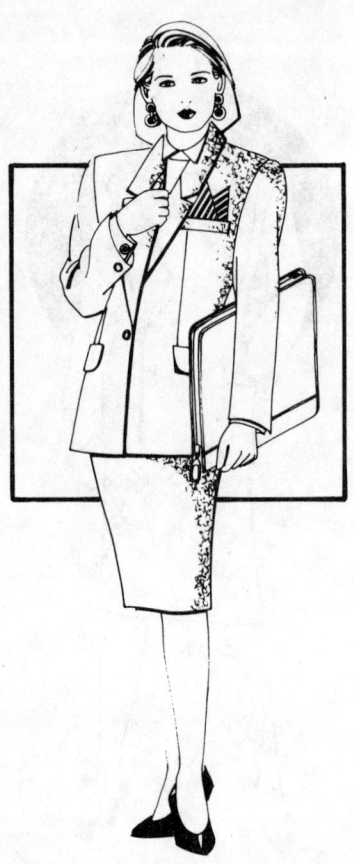

"*When I go for an interview, I'll wear a suit with a comfortable full skirt in case I have to teach a sample lesson. I also wear one piece of expensive jewelry because I don't want them to think I really need this job.*"

Special Education Instructor

"*I would possibly wear an antique stickpin with a scarf, that would be nice, and probably I would pull my hair into a loose bun at the nape of my neck (not the top of my head). I also would make sure my portfolio was attractive and neat both inside and out.*"

Commercial Artist

This is the time to impress people with your competence. Personnel executives, management consultants, and career specialists throughout the country all, for the most part, advocate suits for interviews. To vacillate from the tried and true suit, simply keep in mind the basic qualities that you must convey in this kind of assessment situation: responsibility, self-control, an ability to play that particular game and play it with aplomb. The cosmetic industry might find a woman in an expensive deep purple dress to be wearing the perfect interview outfit, while a managerial position might call for a nubby black-and-white blazer over a black-on-black rayon wrap dress.

Generally it is safest to stay away from extreme statements. However, more creative-based companies may look for you to project a creativity in your attire. It is not an easy trick to look both creative and serious. Again, while picking out something that looks solid, in control, and competent, you still might be very successful in an unmatched suit, a boutique dress with a beautiful shawl, an unmatched suit in ultra-light wool/silk and a hat and gloves, or an ultrasuede long-length skirt with boots and vest.

For a more conservative yet individual touch, go for a vivid pouchette, perhaps a loopy-shaped gold pin, or chain earrings with a bead on the bottom of each chain—something that is a little different, something that expresses what you like. The objective is to stand out from the crowd. You will not do this if you dress "for success" in ultraconservative, mannish attire.

"Color is what works," says one recruiter. "Not just gray or black." Avoid red, however. This still seems just a bit too bold for an interview. Likewise generally avoid chartreuse and fuchsia for all but the most creative situations. Polka dots are a bit high-flying in this setting also and might not make the best first impression, even though in another situation they are terrific.

Women report that when they are interviewed by another woman, they feel they are scrutinized more carefully for what they are wearing, and therefore clothes play a larger part. Women tend to hire the attractive, neatly dressed interviewee who is attractively but conservatively dressed. Keep this in mind if your interviewer is going to be female.

Some Interview Possibilities

- A plum wool coatdress with flecks of black with a lace collar and lace cuffs showing at the sleeves, a deeper plum, multi-accented, double-breasted, padded shoulder jacket with a coordinating silk pocket square, large pearl earrings trimmed with gold.

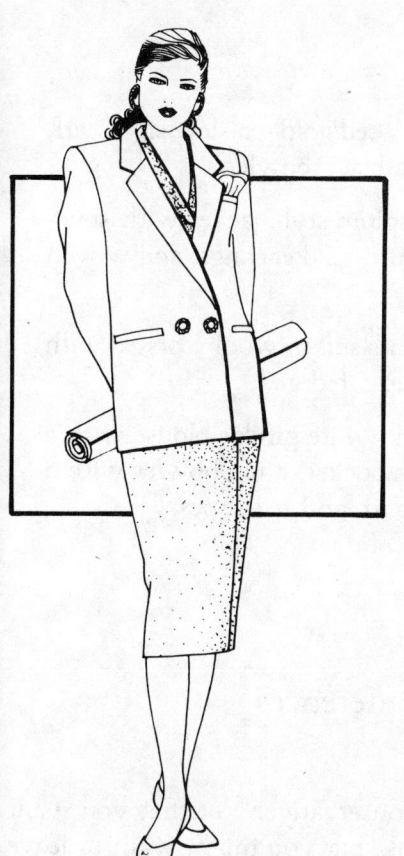

- A beige glen plaid collarless jacket with a solid-brown, pencil-slim skirt, a collarless white silk shirt, a clunky gold necklace, and power pumps in luggage brown.

- A cashmere/silk tweed long-line jacketed suit with a one-tone slim skirt, a full-sleeved silk blouse with matching embroidery on one collar, and hose toned to match the skirt and medium-heel pumps.

- An ultrasuede long-length button-down-the-front skirt with an ultrasuede riding-style jacket, boots, and a silk floral blouse.

- A checked suit with a hand-tooled belt and a lightweight wool sweater with a modified crew neck and embroidered pouchette.

- For the very conservative field, the classic striped cotton shirt with a chalk-striped suit of wool/cashmere and flannel, and bright, contrasting handbag and shoes.

"For interviews, you definitely have to wear a suit."
National Bank Recruiter

Seminars/Brunches

Brunches, conferences, and seminars call for similar approaches no matter the field. You can work in a few "special" touches. For instance, now you can wear a *hat* and probably keep it on. Matching hats, shoes, and gloves make for a very elegant, highly creative look. Possibly a *cape* or a good *coat,* like a cocoon coat, will be noticed. You can wear more interesting combinations and colors, too, like *tweed with lace, red* with *black, plum* with *blue* or *green.*

Some Brunch Possibilities

- A red chemise with black/red/gold paisley silk scarf, black gloves and pumps, a black bowler.

- A fuchsia houndstooth peplum-style jacket with solid-toned slim skirt, bowed shirt, gold earrings, and woven leather gloves.

- Classic bankers'-striped pants suit in wool worsted with silk blouse, high collar, and a fedora.

- A black-checked suit, black/white pindot blouse with a striped pouchette in breast pocket, a red bowler with a black-and-white striped band, and red shoes.

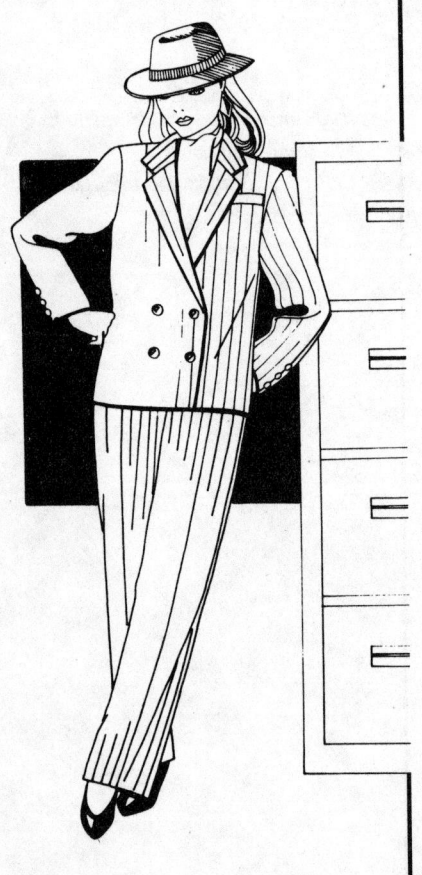

Sales Conferences

These tend to be a bit more conservative. Not that you want to revert to the corporateer look, but you might want to leave the red-and-black paisley at home.

Stick to subtle-toned suits, classy gold accessories, and not too much jewelry. If your company is ultraconservative, as many still are, you may have to create your own version of navy over pale blue.

- A navy wool crepe dropped-waist suit with a large single waist button, powder-blue silk wrap blouse, and a large gold lapel pin.

- A navy-and-white checked jacket with a slim navy wool skirt, and a blue-and-white-striped crisp cotton shirt.

- A navy/ice-striped suit with a collarless blue silk shirt, and a clunky gold necklace.

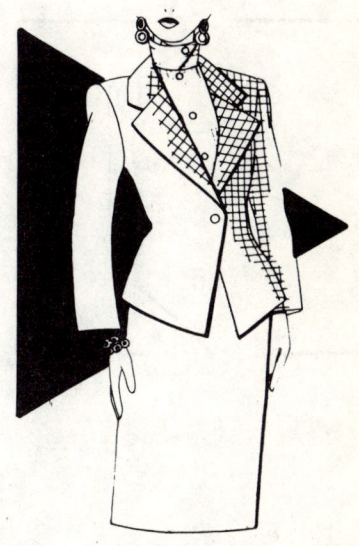

Picnics and Outings

This is where you can relax a bit, indulge yourself in color and show even more personal flair. It's also a big area of concern for most women. When does casual become too casual? How much skin can safely be revealed? Is there a rule of thumb to make choices easier? Yes.

Generally speaking, if you're worried about whether a garment is too bare, it probably is. The impression to convey is that you are ready for chic, formal pleasantries, like something out of an F. Scott Fitzgerald novel. You want to look ready for fun but not a zoo outing with your children.

Picnic attire could be a skirt or pants with a washed silk shirt and possibly a jacket. Pants in a soft, pleated style, worn with a large gold-buckled suede belt, a floral silk jacket and huge and colorful yet classy earrings is beautiful business picnic attire. If jumpsuits appeal to you, now is the time to wear them, especially if they come with a matching jacket. A fabric such as rayon seersucker looks quite cool yet elegant in a summer jumpsuit. Another sensational outfit would be a vivid overblouse with a multicolored floral-print skirt, both in washed silk.

Also for an afternoon business gathering in the out-of-doors, try a twill dock short (just above the knee) outfit with a classic

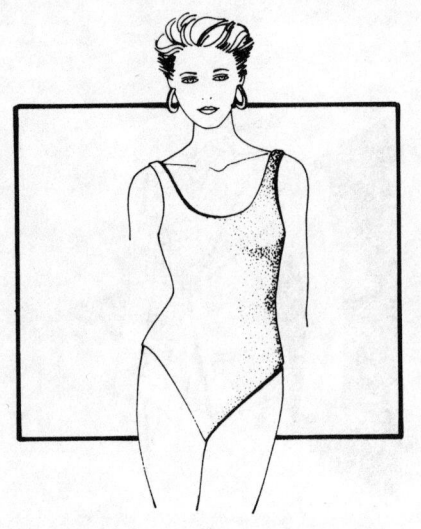

crew neck, a gold monogrammed "T," and perhaps a nautical windbreaker also in white twill. And bring out the Porsche or retro-sunglasses.

You might also want to wear a colorful gaucho skirt with a stretchy belt, a bright shirt, and a quilted cropped jacket for a playful yet highly stylish appearance. With something this dramatic, wear only bold earrings.

Low-heeled skimmers are fine with these fashions, as are woven leather sling-back flats. Or with jumpsuits or pants, you might also wear a nice low-heeled but comfortable pump in a bright blue or red with a snap-on grosgrain ornament.

As for swimsuits, the classic tank is a good bet. To keep it from boring you totally, select one in beautiful stained-glass multitones and wear a wrap, floral tunic over it; or choose a front-lace tank in polka dots with a huge white cotton cardigan with matching dots. High-cut suits which show a lot of thigh are fine for Club Med but not the company outing.

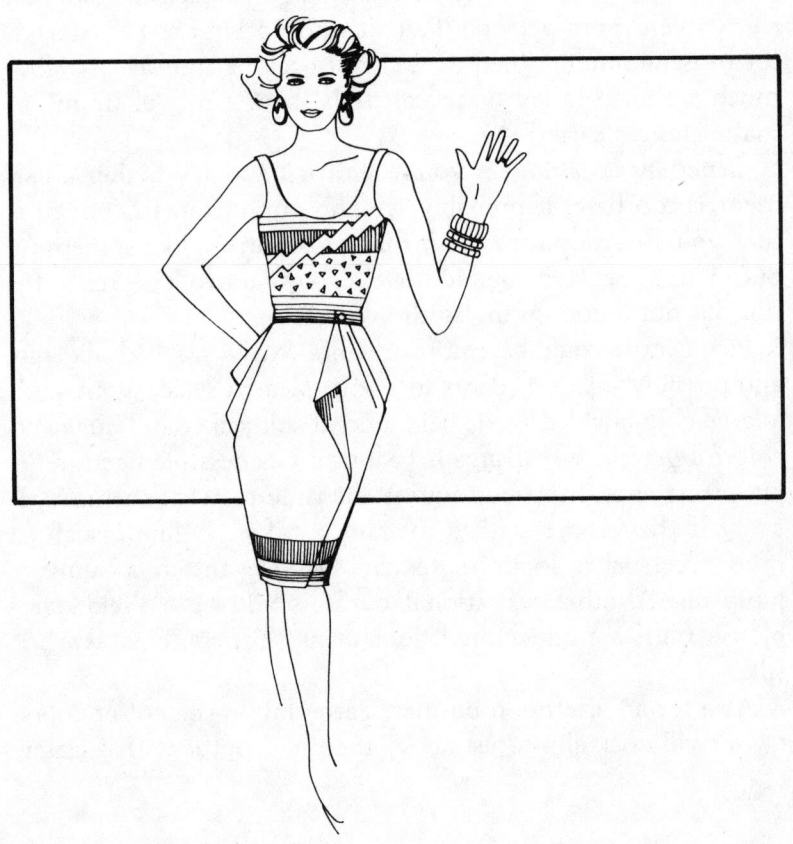

Cotton is a fabric that does play a role now in casual yet good-quality shirts and skirts, as, for example, with an unlined, cotton blazer or cardigan. Think of Ralph Lauren and you probably have the right outdoor look to convey quality, responsibility, and fun at the same time.

An unfettered, flowing batik-print cotton dress with a long full skirt is a colorful, relatively casual look that suits the greater freedom of picnics or casual company outings.

As for what to wear over the bathing suit while you're getting to the pool or water's edge, wrap skirts that tie on are very good, as is a huge scarf tied sarong style.

You probably won't want to wear hose. So what then? Pants offer one solution. Knee-high hose or argyles are another option. Bare legs may be all right if they are not pasty white, and short-term tanning makeup can make this option more agreeable.

You will still want to accessorize with casual wear. Bracelets appear in this fashion; sport and fun watches become prominent. Huge earrings are appropriate and fun as well.

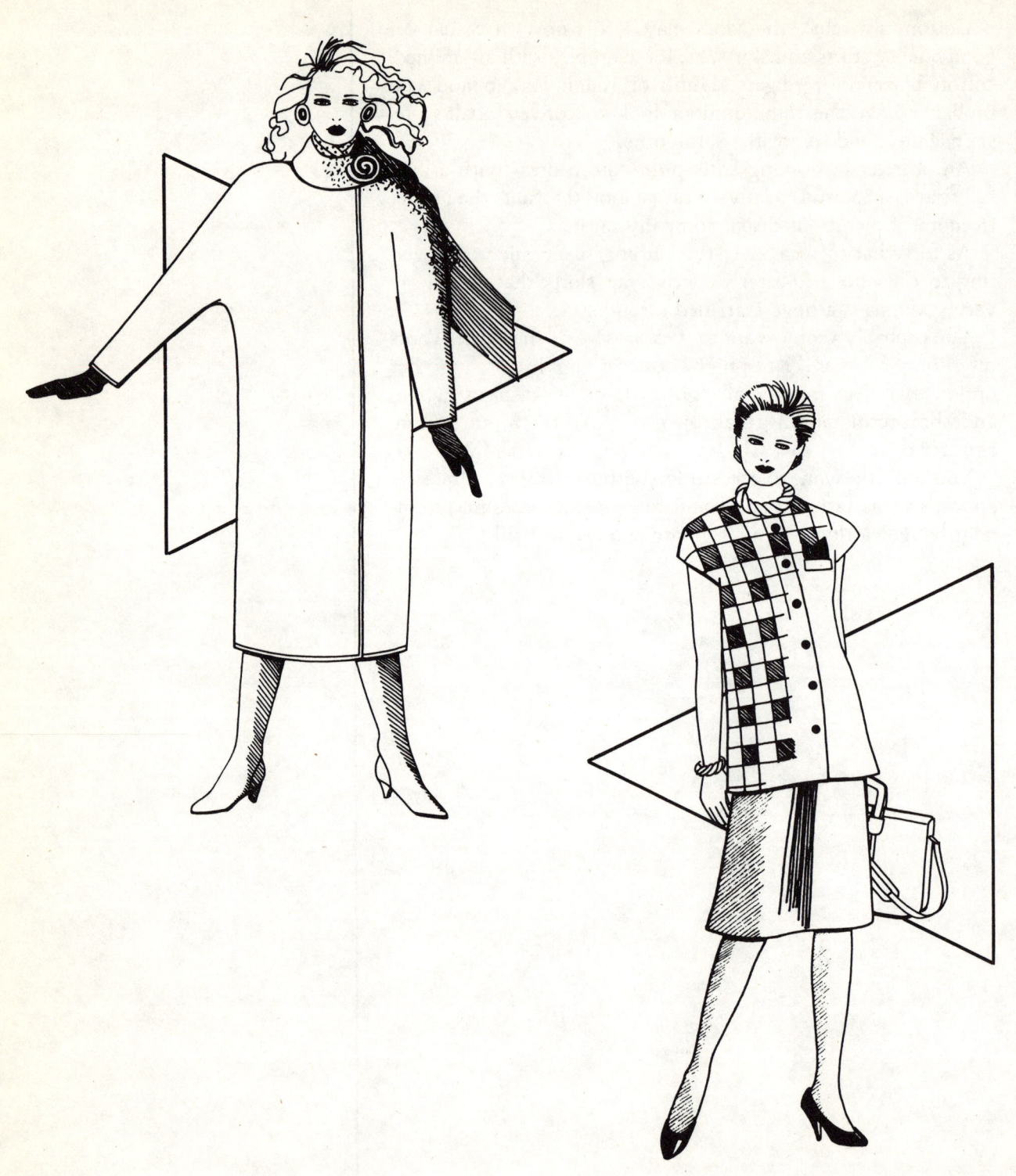

Pregnant with Style

You can retain your business and feminine persona while pregnant. The same basic principles for businesswear outlined in this book will still apply nicely with just a few "alterations" in approach. In fact, you don't have to buy an entirely new wardrobe; it makes sense to buy only a few choice items that will take you through the five to six months looking great.

The question is, should your goal be to hide your pregnant appearance? The answer is a qualified no. To hide anything that obvious is impossible. What you should do, however, is keep your pregnancy from interfering with your business image. This chapter offers basic hints for helping you keep your business savoir-faire just a little bit more obvious than your impending motherhood.

"If I concentrated on slim, short skirts, and big bulky tops, either blouses or jackets, I found that a lot of people didn't really even notice that I was pregnant. Especially if I wore bright jewelry."
Accounting VP

Maternity Takes a Back Seat

Rather than run out in the first rush of excitement and buy everything new at an expectant mothers' shop, first go through your closet. The clothes you buy in the first throes of preg-

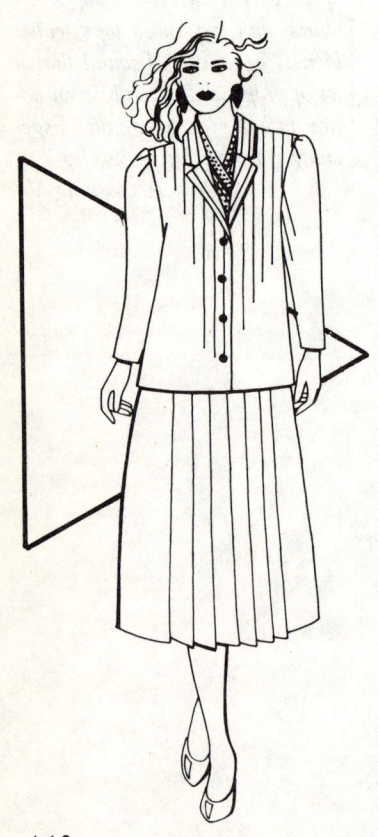

nancy passion may not suit you or the weather when you are ready to slip them on, so it is best to buy maternity fashions frugally. The first three months you can wear your own clothes. Months four to nine are the problem area.

Evaluating Your Closet

Consider the seasons in which you will be showing. This should determine how far you have to stretch your wardrobe.

Eliminate skirts without elasticized waists because you won't be able to wear them after the third month or so. Also eliminate all fitted jackets from your planning. For now you must content yourself with roomy, bulky fashions.

Look for loose and cardigan-shaped jackets in your closet and pull them out. They can be used as basic pieces.

Analyze your choices and narrow down to a few colors what you intend to interweave in your nine-month fashion plans. After you have done this, and the third month is just about over, it's time to shop and fill in the gaps.

Shopping

Certainly you should make the rounds of maternity specialty shops. Some do cater to the executive woman and tend to carry some sophisticated fashions—not the more typical "precious" fare. But don't avoid your usual small shops or the women's section in department stores. They can offer infinite possibilities!

- Try to stay within your size, because to go beyond it in order to expand a waistline will probably mean drooping, sagging necklines and in general a contribution to the notion that pregnant women inevitably look sloppy.

- Look for basic skirts and tops. Keep watch for big, easy tops and elasticized skirts that just might carry you through. If you have no jackets that you can use, look for an appropriate shapeless style. Do not buy a jacket that cuts off at the waistline, as this will fast be vanishing and anything that emphasizes this area will not be attractive. Basically you want to dress simply, with no breaks in clothing at the waist, working for a smooth silhouette from neck to hem. Long-line jackets will work best throughout the pregnancy and still give you lots of wear after the baby arrives!

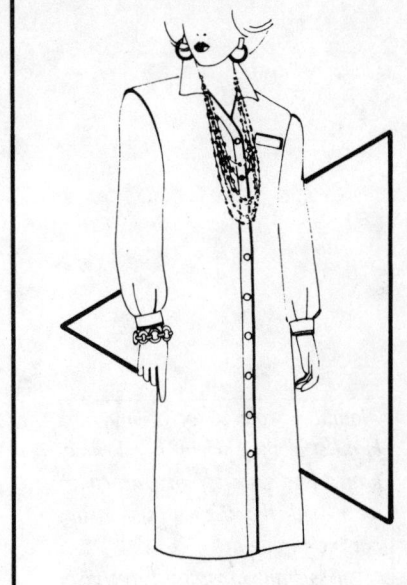

- Loose or waistless dresses in non-clingy fabrics are a great option. A loose-fitting chemise with full sleeves, notched collar in perhaps a stripe will look fine during and after pregnancy. Wrap dresses, blouses, and coats are perfect for this time. You can even go to short hems (no higher than skimming the knee) to emphasize the slenderness of your legs. Coatdresses are a good choice but not in a paisley or large print. Small prints tend to become "cutesy" under these circumstances, too, and so it is best to keep coatdresses or any other kind of dress in simple, elegant, solid colors. Go for smooth, unbroken silhouettes.

  Lines of packaged garments available in better stores include such things as kimono coats, matching elastic-waist skirts, tunic tops, and more, all labeled "one-size-fits-all." Depending on your field, you could design some easy to wear and attractive outfits for yourself. Kimonos with some Oriental details worn over a black dress can be very pretty. This, too, is actually part of power dressing, in that you don't have to show up in pinstripes.

  Styles to avoid are the "earth mother" type or anything labeled "efficient," "indispensable," or "casually affordable."

  No doubt there will come a point when you must purchase some maternity wear. The only rule here is to try to draw attention away from the obvious. Interesting earrings, a fabulous necklace, and maternity choices that are simple and subtle in color are your best bets.

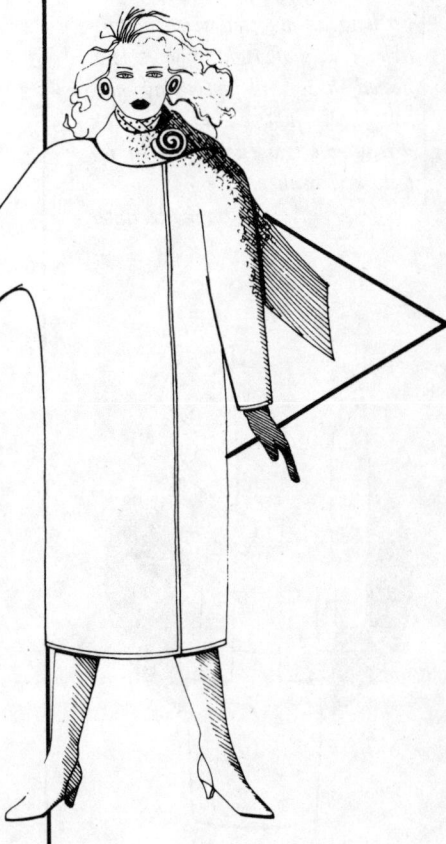

- Wintertime? You have to think about a coat, unless you have a nice tent-style or Ottoman wool cocoon in the closet—chic, stylish, and all-encompassing. Do not buy a maternity coat as they generally are less well made than regular ones. If you must make a coat purchase, shop the regular section of the store and select a roomy coat that will look good no matter the size of your girth.

A cape will be perfect now and can be worn later, too. Unfortunately, capes are not as warm as button-up coats, but with the right garments underneath, such as a heavy sweater or a wool serge suit, the cape can work beautifully and look smashing. Your body temperature will generally run higher than normal now anyway from carrying extra, unaccustomed weight, so even one of your regular winter coats left mostly unbuttoned, with warm garments underneath, should be sufficient.

- Toward the end of the third month, buy shoes with no more than a two-inch heel. By attempting to balance on high heels, you can aggravate your back which is always working overtime to keep you upright. The ideal shoe is a low-heeled skimmer, with an added touch such as a grosgrain bow or a flower at the toe. Because your feet may swell, the shoes will get hard wear, so don't pay as much for them as you would normally.

Most people expect pregnant women to look less than fashionable, so any successful efforts you make will be well received. Those impressions last well beyond your time of pregnancy.

Accessories

Accessories become very important now, especially around the face, neck, and arms. So this is the time to indulge yourself in earrings, necklaces, bracelets, and a gorgeous watch.

Wear belts low slung to the fifth or sixth month. Short women, however, should not wear belts low on their stomach, as it will further minimize their height.

Shawls, hats, and jewelry, dark-toned hose and shoes, bags, and gloves are all accessories that play a big part in getting you through pregnancy in a chic way. They convey an attitude that says, "I am in control of my life." Not vice versa.

Then accessorize (without overdoing) to create a fashion look. Colors will help a great deal, so by all means indulge in brightly colored shirts and pocket squares.

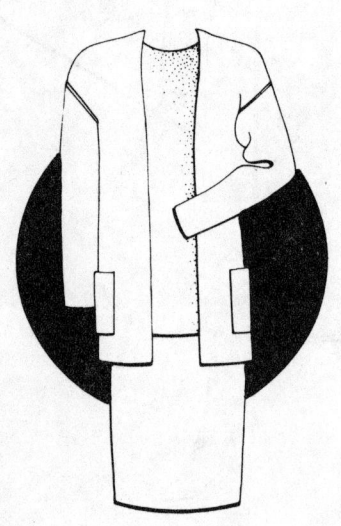

Three Types

Classic with a Twist

- A brown/black striped collarless, buttonless loose jacket with huge patch pockets over a cowl-neck brown over-shirt, worn over loose-fitting pants, with brown-toned hose and gold jewelry.

- A gray plaid capped-sleeve top over a short black slim skirt with black hose, two-inch heeled spectator power pumps, a silver sculpted necklace with black beads, and silver earrings.

- A fingertip-length jacket in gray flannel, no collar, with a slim plaid skirt.

- A red free-flowing dress with a black collar, black buttons, and a black/white silk pocket pouchette.

- A shawl-collared cardigan jacket in black with shoulder pads and huge buttons, a slim skirt, and an antique neck brooch.

- A short-cut bolero jacket (falling just below the bust-line) over a black wedge-shaped chemise.

- A navy-checked double-breasted jacket and skirt with a bowed blouse, crystal drop earrings, and a navy hat with a red band.

Avant-Garde

- A soft wool boucle onyx jacket, a skirt with gold buttons, and a huge stole in the same fabric.

- A bright stained-glass patterned roomy top over a soft, full skirt, with a foulard-collared jacket, colored crystal beads, and matching long earrings.

- A swirling silk scarf of many satin-striped colors in houndstooth, wrapped around one shoulder over a black dress with clunky gold jewelry.

- A fuchsia long-line collarless jacket, over a pink over-

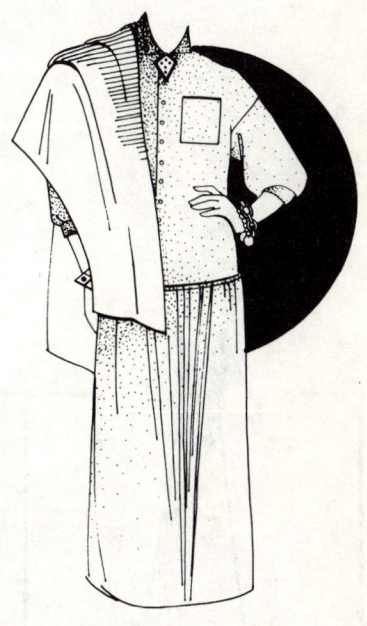

size silk top and a fuchsia skirt, pale-pink hose, and pink shoes with flower clips.

- Over a purple chemise, the drape of a huge classic cover-up jersey ruana fastened with a large gold pin at the shoulder.

- A boxy-jacketed suit with a velvet French sailor's cap and white gloves.

- A classic all-black suit with flower clip buttons and huge pearl earrings encircled with rhinestones.

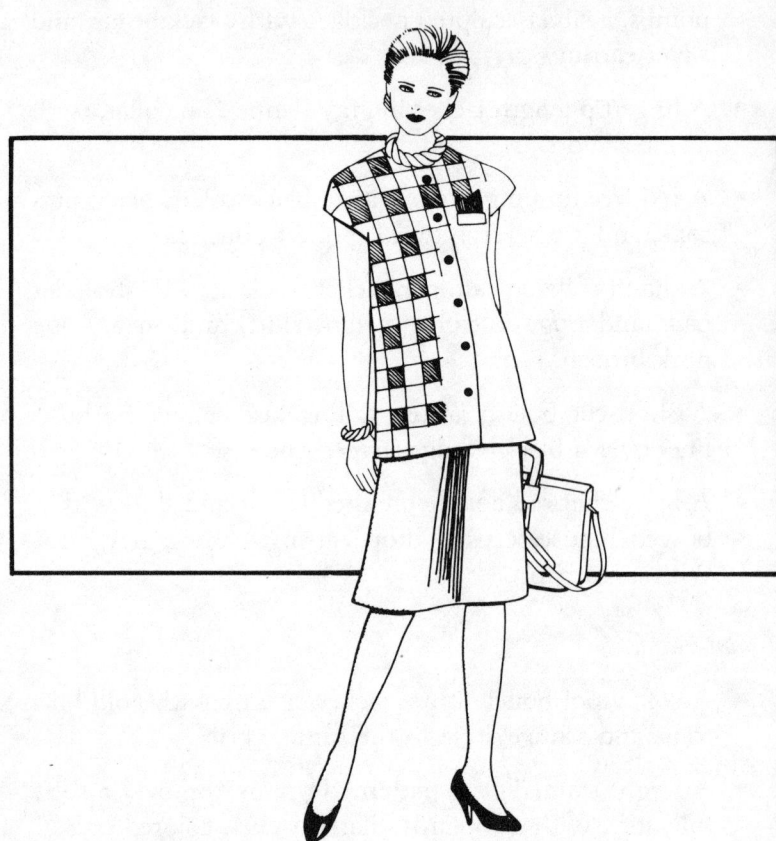

Exotic

- Rows and rows of long pearl strands over a red-and-black checked soft wrap maternity dress and a red loose-fitting jacket.

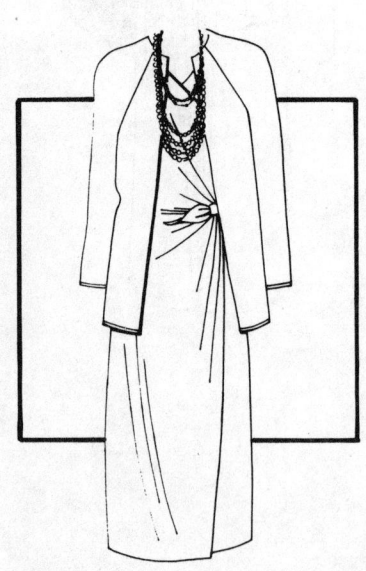

- A pindot chemise with kickpleat of polka dots. Wear with a polka-dot neck scarf.

- A loose-fitting soft dress with a tie belt worn just below the waist, and a contrasting bowler hat with matching power pumps.

- A red-and-black plaid cardigan-style loose jacket with black wool soft-styled slacks, huge gold earrings, and a mock turtleneck top.

- With a dashing white full-sleeved blouse, wear a huge sweater vest in red or apple green, and a cream wool skirt.

- A plaid long-line black/white jacket with a small checked black/white skirt and black-and-white pindot overblouse, with black earrings.

- A rose-print overblouse with puffed sleeves and a jewel neck with a classic black suit and huge gold earrings.

- A paisley extra long, extra loose one-button jacket over solid-tone colors with a contrasting paisley shawl or an antique pin.

Dos and Don'ts

Do

Wear tops out. Tuck them in, and you cut your look in half and come across looking merely fat instead of pregnant.

Wear a dark top on the outside with a loose checked jacket (a jacket creates a vertical line, which can trick people into thinking you do not have a stomach) and a dark skirt.

Go for brights, that's right, bright colors in tops, such as forest green, purple, fuchsia, all those colors that you've heard pregnant women shouldn't wear.

Give yourself freedom to explore new possibilities such as kimonos or tunic tops. A short washed-silk kimono tied with a scarf over pull-on washed-silk pants, accessorized with gold earrings is a beautiful look.

Try long-line sweaters. Geometric prints are quite chic.

Elasticized blouson tops work very well and can be used to hide an elasticized waistband. Go for patterns in purses and shoes.

Choose slim-line skirts, not full, looser looks.

Don't

Try to wear your regular clothes after they have become too tight.

Allow yourself to look messy in any way. This is the time to look neat above all.

Wear in excess such things as large floral prints, plaids, dots, or stripes.

Try for glamour over comfort. See if you can make the two work together, rather than sacrifice one for the other.

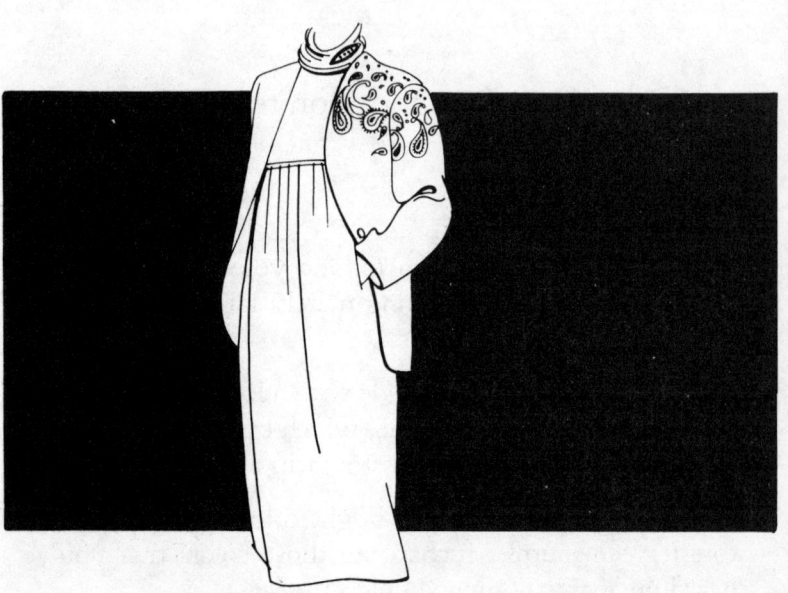

Hold back on your fashion imagination during this time. There is plenty you can do to look femininely businesslike during your expectancy.

Ignore small details such as nail polish, hats, silky fabrics, or hair bows. Motherhood does not mean you have to give these up.

Think you can't stay up-to-date.

Overspend on maternity clothes.

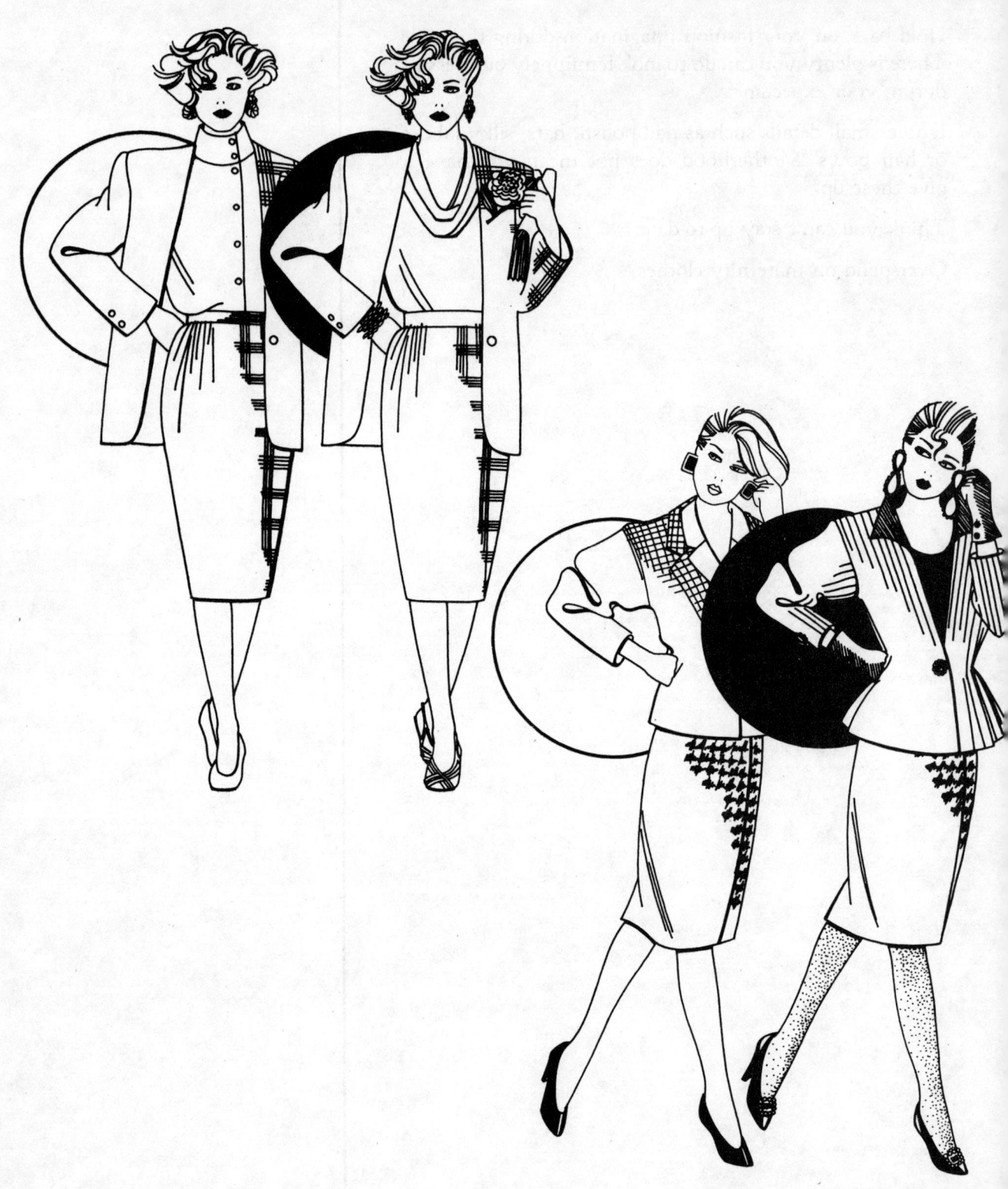

Day Into Night

Probably the most exciting effects come from transformations as in the caterpillar's metamorphosis into the butterfly. While none of us walks around looking like a caterpillar at work, we definitely do maintain a humbler look than when appearing at a dinner engagement. Thus the change from day to night can prove a dramatic one.

To reveal the backstage workings of this drama, we have selected three classic professional daytime outfits: an unmatched suit with a checked jacket and houndstooth wrap skirt, a glen plaid collarless suit, and a silk sheath dress. We have taken these basic business looks and turned them into evening business attire by both adding and subtracting. Largely, the secret is in the accessories, employing with imagination such things as scarves, belts, earrings, necklaces, stockings, and shoes. But some looks also profit by substitution of one item for another, one type of jacket for another.

Voilà. Daytime career chic turns into nighttime career glamour. Nothing overwhelming, nothing sexy. Still, femininity and attractiveness keep their place in the transition from sunshine to moonlight.

The following are some suggestions for ways in which these basic outfits can be transformed.

> "To go from day to night, I add jewelry or a scarf with a shot of gold, or maybe an unusual belt with a brilliant buckle. I keep special makeup at work to get ready for an evening meeting; blush with a little sparkle for example."
>
> *Financial Analyst*

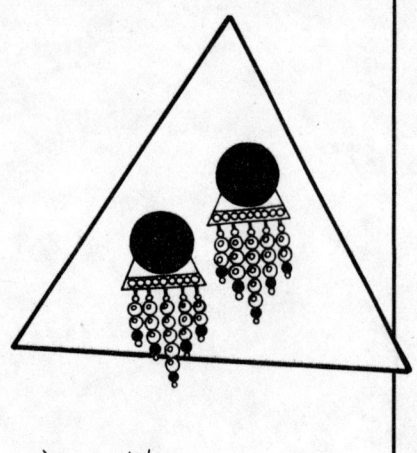

The Unmatched Suit

- Replace the jacket altogether with a satin cream-and-black pin-striped jacket with a peplum, a single button at the waist, and a black tuxedo-style collar. Replace the daytime blouse with a black silk chemise underneath the jacket. Exchange the daytime gold pin for large black pearl earrings in an elaborate setting and wear these with the black chemise. Take off those suntan-toned hose and substitute black sheer hose and higher-heeled black silk pumps. Wear a rhinestone buckle on the toe of each shoe.

- Clip a cricket—those rosette clips—over each jacket button to change it instantly to a dressier effect. Instead of the wrap skirt, put on a black silk pencil-slim skirt. Wear a gold satin rope belt with ornaments. Carry a small black silk handbag and wear black gloves. Add a black hair bow.

- Wear a soft cashmere sweater and just a stole—no jacket with the houndstooth skirt. Sometimes getting away from the "suit look" alone makes an outfit look dressier. Wear sparkling jet earrings in an exotic shape. Add a belt with a bold, gold buckle with rows of gold chains attached.

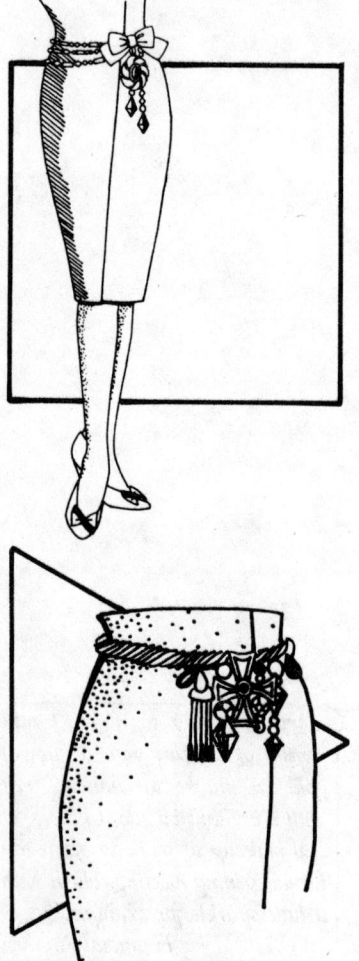

The Silk Sheath Dress

- Remove the daytime jacket you were wearing with

this dress. Add rows and rows of rose quartz beads. Take off daytime scarf to bare the neck.

- Or add a three-tiered gold chain belt.

- Or put a bow clip with rhinestones on plain pumps with higher heels.

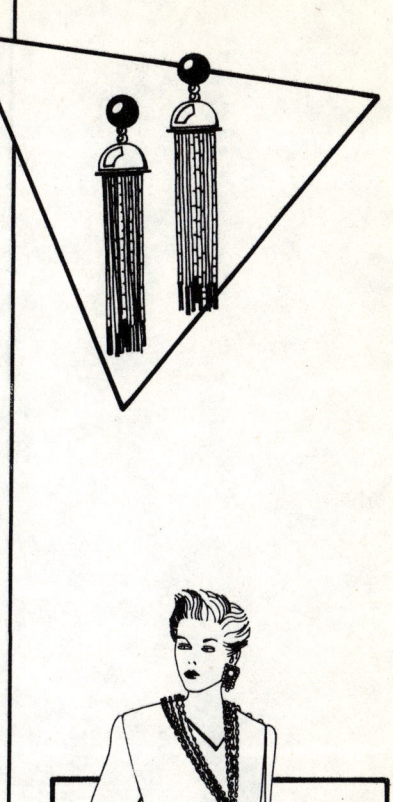

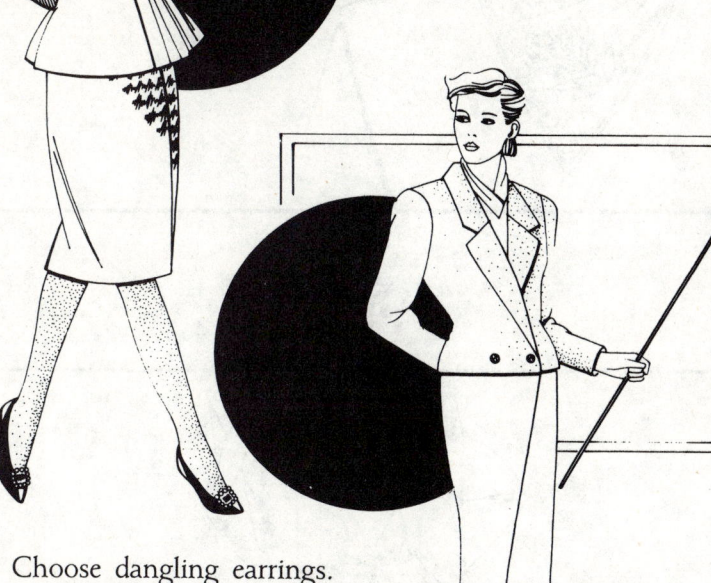

- Choose dangling earrings. Now you can go all out. Stash those more conservative baubles in the office closet drawer. Wrap a Spanish-style lightweight wool stole with a long fringe around your shoulders and pin it with a sparkling rhinestone antique brooch.

- Wear an antique rhinestone pin on one side or at the center of the neck with a chiffon floral scarf wrapped round and round.

- Wear a silk jacket in contrasting stripe and wear with

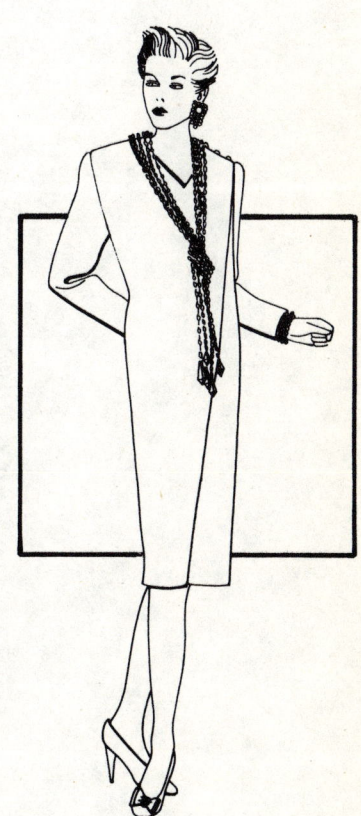

a dressy bow in the hair. Add a stretchy gold belt, along with a Greek gold-coin necklace.

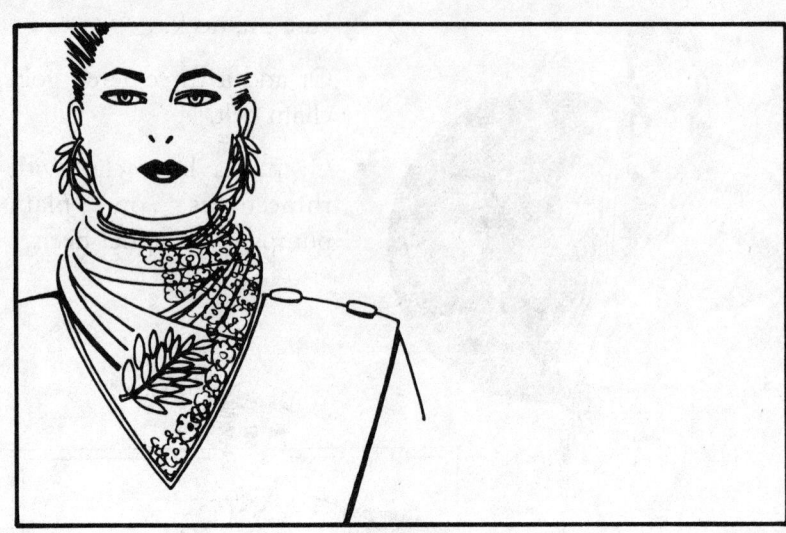

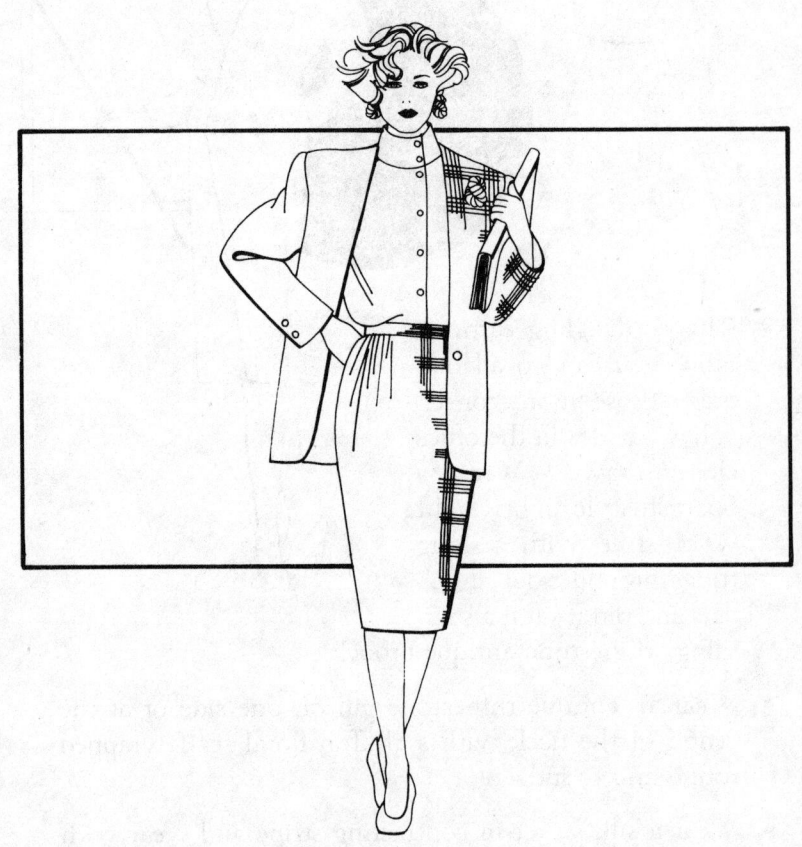

The Glen Plaid Suit

- Exchange the gold pin for a many-rowed pearl choker. Exchange the daytime white blouse for a lush, soft cashmere sweater. Change from suntan-toned pantyhose to smokey tones. It is possible to wear high-heeled sandals now.

- Drape a cream silk scarf around your neck and fasten with an antique gold brooch with many colored stones. Put on high-heeled patent pumps and slip those lower-heeled spectators into the office closet.

- Add a gold-and-pearl pendant and drape a handwoven Peruvian stole over your shoulders. Leave the briefcase or the tote behind, and carry a small silk purse with a pearl clip.

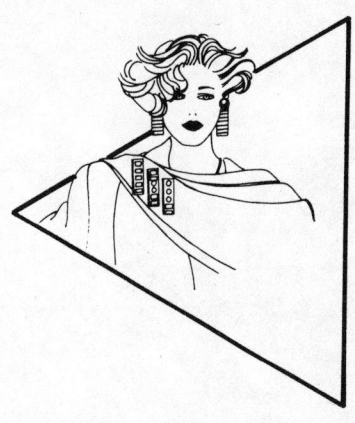

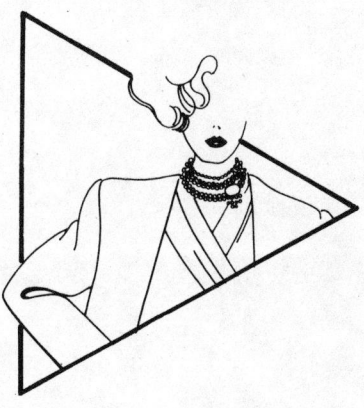

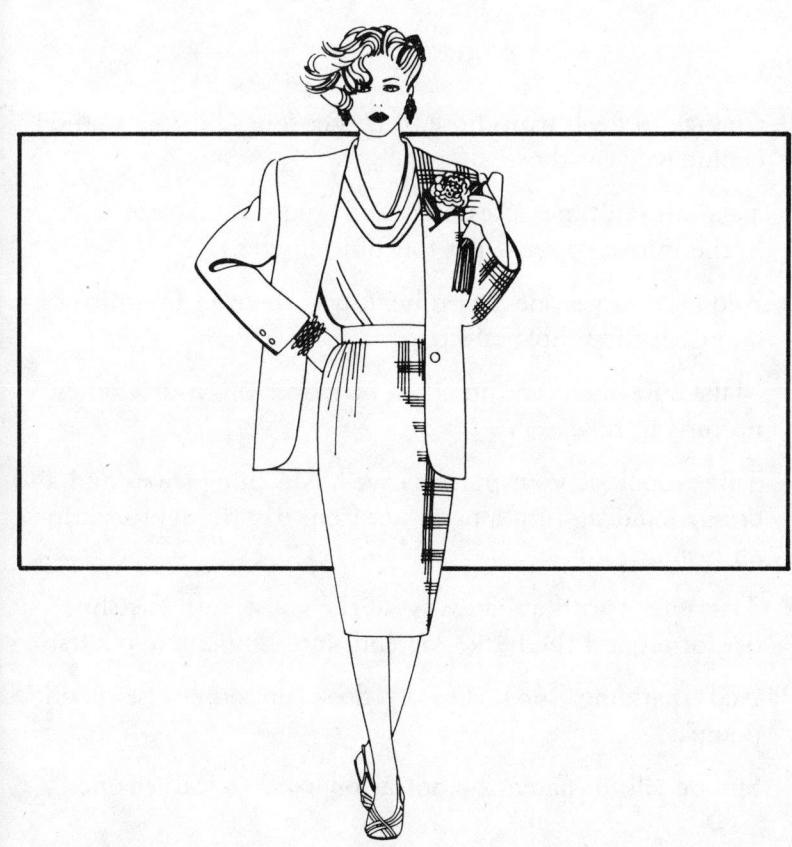

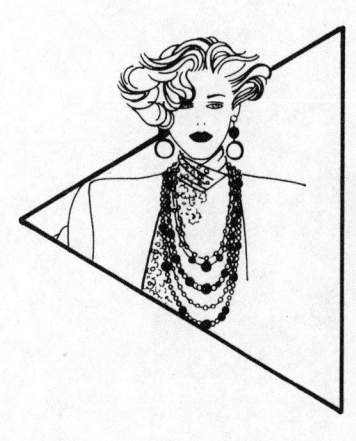

- Put on a lacy blouse and accompany this with many rows of long, long beads. Pick up the glitter in large earrings and add a grosgrain bow to the toe of each high-heeled shoe.

- Wrap your hair up and fasten it with an antique, faux-gem comb. Take off the high-neck daytime blouse and instead wear a scoop-neck silk blouse in a vivid color. Add a huge, floppy flower pin at one shoulder of the jacket, or clip it over a front waist button.

- Add white silk gloves, a white silk scarf, huge gold earrings and higher-heeled, silk shoes with gold button clips.

Dos and Don'ts

Do

Change to fresh pantyhose. If darker tones fit your outfit, definitely wear those.

Take off daytime accessories and study your basic outfit in the mirror to see what touch it requires.

Add accessories one at a time. Study them in the mirror, taking in the whole effect.

Make sure there are no spots or marks on your clothes, no runs in hose.

Take a look at your purse as well. Matching shoes and a dressy handbag turn a basic suit from day to nightwear in an instant.

Try tying a scarf a new way, at the waist, over the shoulder, or around the neck. Tie ends into flower-like pouffs.

Add sparkling shoe clips to dress up otherwise plain pumps.

Slip on silk or patent pumps as opposed to leather ones.

Don't

Wait until that night at five o'clock to figure out what to wear.

Overdramatize or over-accessorize.

Go sexy which means revealing, low-cut, mini, or tight.

Wear fancy diamond earrings with a glen plaid, houndstooth, or color-layered look.

Try to dress up a manstyle pin-striped suit with chiffon scarves. Stick to a more subdued effect of Italian silk paisley with fringes.

Wear a silk camisole without a jacket. It's just a little too bare.

Overdo on perfume.

Forget that the look must still convey business *over* pleasure.

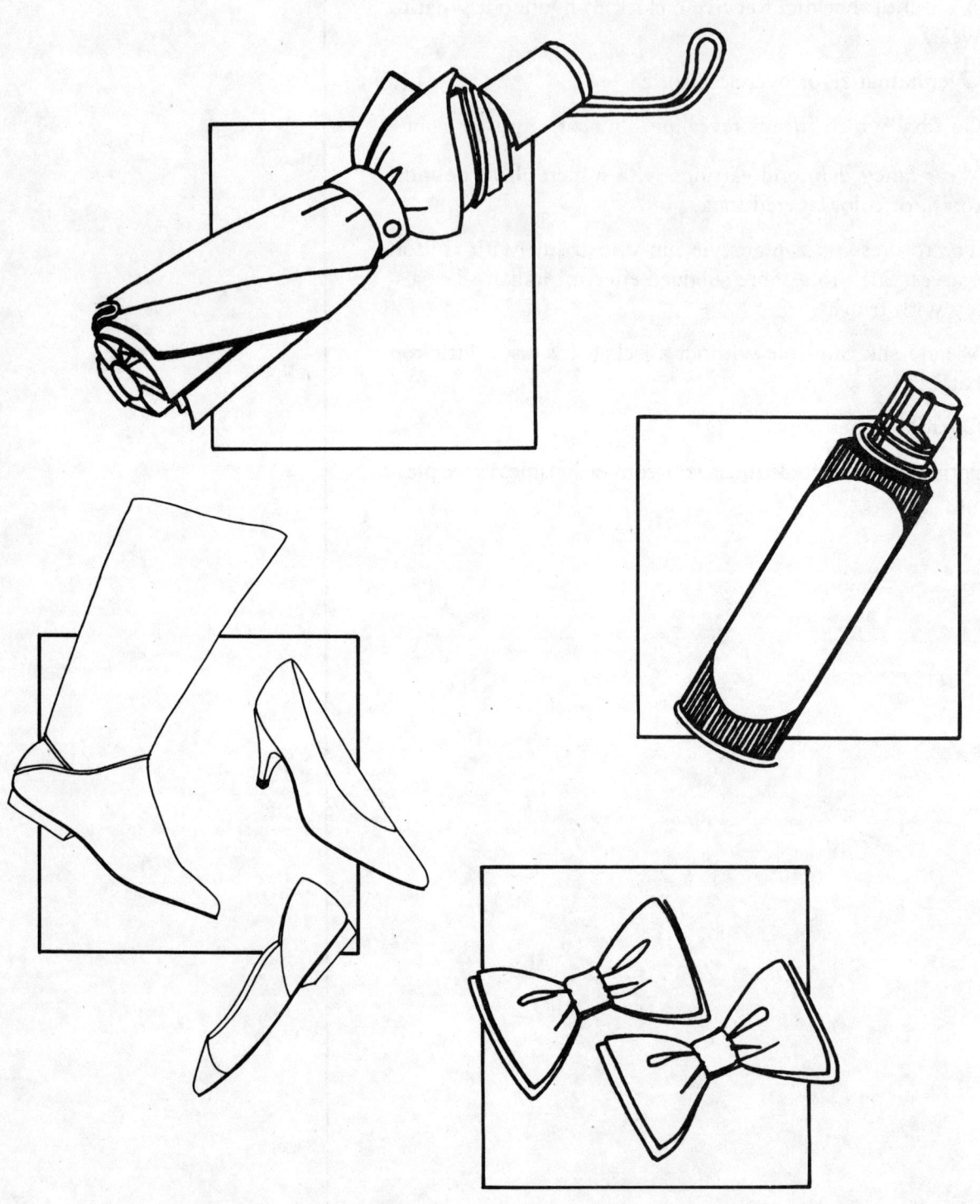

CHAPTER

9

The Office Closet

The office "closet" is where you keep things for freshening up, that extra "exec" touch, and basic metamorphosing. You will always want to be prepared for a sudden meeting, a surprise boardroom appearance, or nighttime dinners feting a client or welcoming a partner to town. For this reason there are a lot of items that are smart to keep on hand.

Being organized can turn the office closet into an efficient support supply for a fashionable working image.

There are two functions for the office closet: 1) getting those practical but necessary items out of sight so that the decor around you is not brought down by them, and 2) storing things that will allow you to glide smoothly from one situation to another throughout a demanding day.

Where to put everything is the first and key question. Do you have a hook behind your door? A jacket hanging over an umbrella hanging underneath a coat, scarf, and hat plus gloves can look messy. If you hold a private conference and need to close your door, suddenly, a rod full of clothes swings past.

Do you kick extra shoes underneath the desk? They can be seen, there, you know, from the other side if, like most desks, yours does not come all the way to the floor. The sight of shoes lying about does not look efficient or businesslike.

Do you stick everything in one jumbled drawer which you

must rifle through whenever you need nail polish or a pair of pantyhose? Where do you leave your rain or snow boots? What *do* you do with your umbrella, and where do you keep the accessories, purse, gloves, scarves, that you need to have on hand for dinner occasions?

Some women do set aside a spare drawer for their "closet," some use the backs of their doors, some, however, commandeer a company locker, and some refuse to keep clothing at work and instead dress for the day that morning and carry along whatever they might need in a tote. If something unexpected comes up later, they dash home. It's an arrangement that is called "making do" and is awkward as well as inefficient.

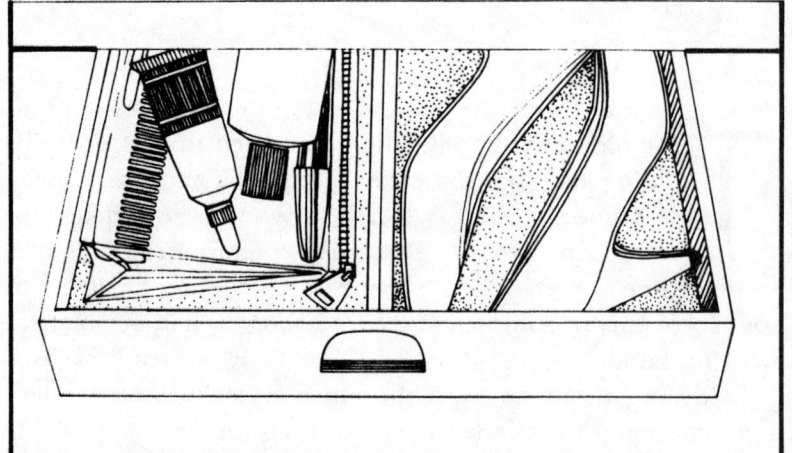

The best way is to find adequate space in a locker or closet, away from your desk and your work space. This presupposes that your company will or can supply such a place. If they do, use it. If not, use a drawer for small items such as a toiletries bag filled with miniatures, and purchase a nondescript garment bag to hang on the back of your door. Place your spare blouse or jacket inside (you could also use the bag pockets for small items) and keep it zipped up. The look is clean and visitors will think you're prepared for a business trip.

The contents of your office closet will vary according to your own particular needs. Some women might keep fingernail glue while others store crackers for a late afternoon energy sag.

Certain universals, however, do apply. Umbrellas, for instance, should be kept at the office for those days when rain doesn't threaten in the morning, yet surprises everyone around the end of the day. Rain shoes or rubber boots might also be kept on hand under the same rationale.

One pair of pantyhose in every color you typically wear is an essential item. Walking around the office with a run in a stocking is definitely not a look you want to be stuck with all day!

If you walk to work in sneakers, keep them out of sight during the day. If you wear walking shoes in inclement weather, stow them in the closet, too. Nothing should be left to show from around or underneath your desk.

Hats, wool scarves, gloves, and any shopping bags should be shut away out of sight.

Some items to include in the office closet:

- Umbrella

- Two to three pairs of pantyhose

- Silk chemise or dressy blouse (for evening changes)

- Foul weather shoes or boots

- Rain hat

- Handkerchief (2)

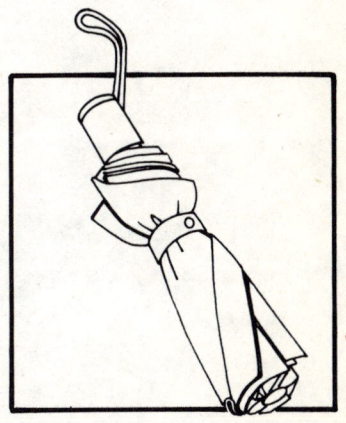

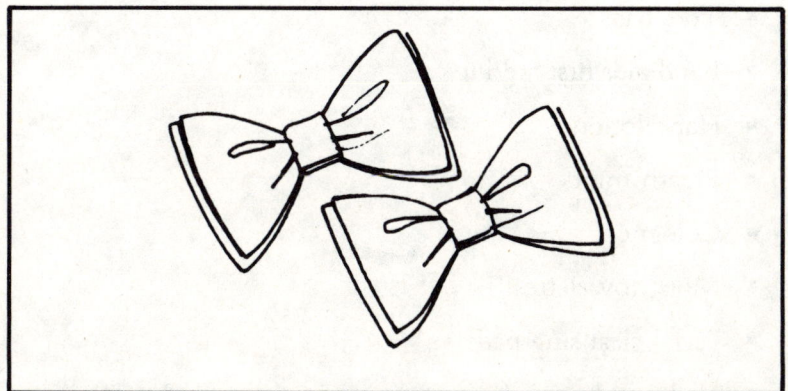

- Travel iron
- Light-wool challis stole for evening

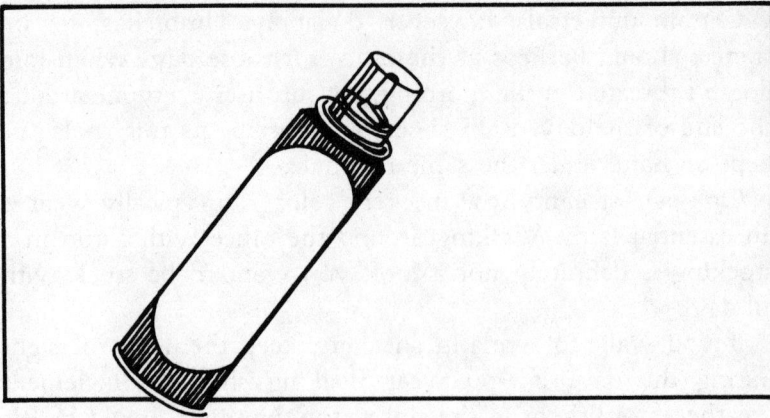

- Dressy earrings (for day to night transformation)
- Dressy shoe clips (for evening changes)
- Silk or chiffon scarf in a print which goes with one of your basic colors
- Flower pin
- Hand mirror with magnifying glass on one side/regular on the other
- Comb, brush, and hair ornaments and styling helps
- Emery boards
- Eyeglasses/sunglasses
- Tote bag
- Band aids/first-aid kit
- Hand lotion
- Breath mints
- Cologne
- Moist towelettes
- Facial cleansing pads
- Nail polish, polish remover, and fingernail glue
- Spot remover
- Baby powder for removing grease spots

- Small sewing kit with pins
- Aspirins
- Stocking mender
- Deodorant
- Toothbrush/paste/dental floss

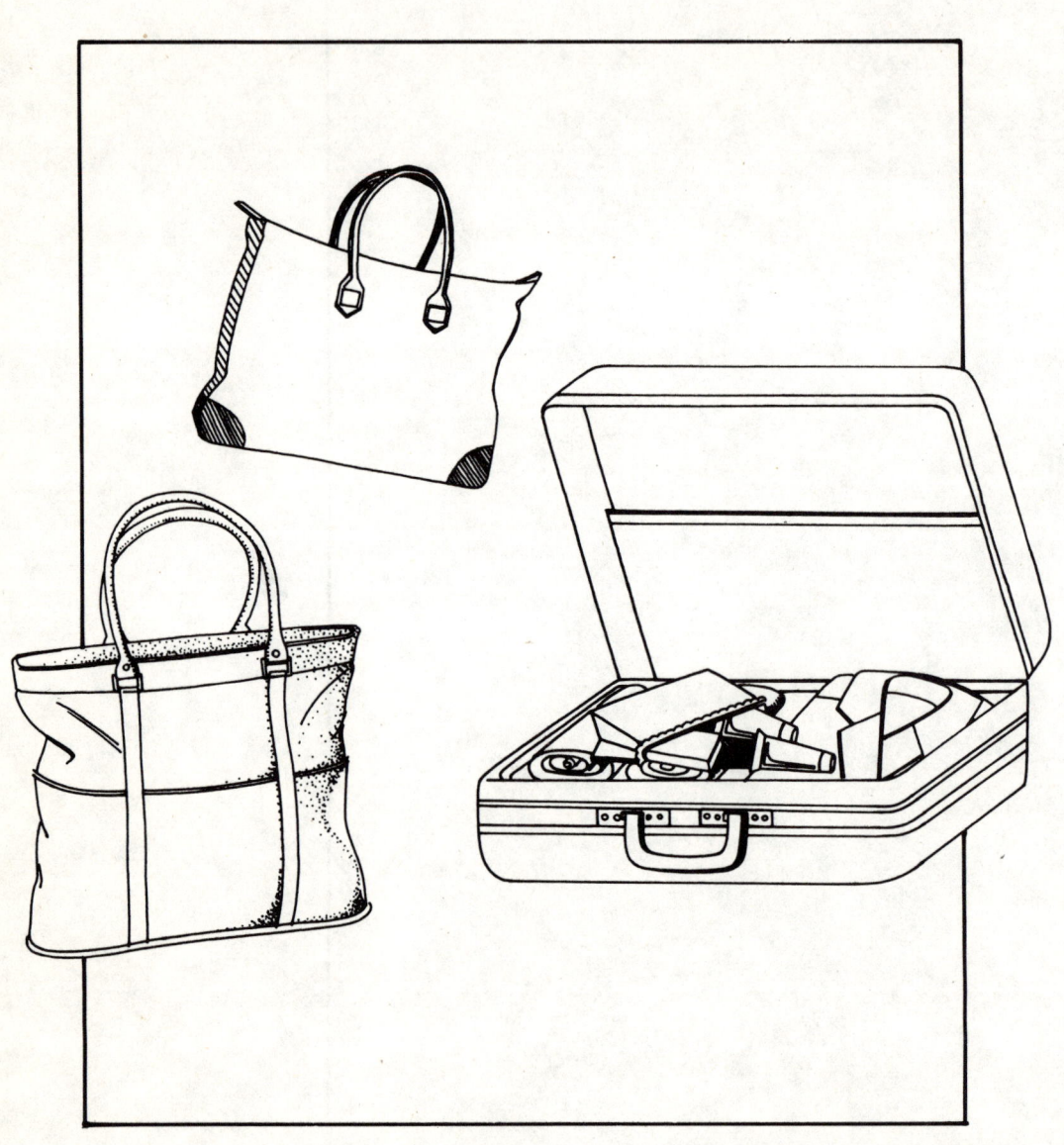

Traveling with Ease

Conferences, conventions, and presentations frequently mean travel. If you're going to be met by a business associate, you obviously can't wear jeans on the plane. Thus you are faced with the question of how to feel comfortable for hours en route, and yet look chic upon arrival. And, as if that were not enough of a dilemma, there is still the matter of retaining your femininity while underlining your professional persona. It's a tall order, but here are some ways to present just the right attractive and unrumpled picture with only a bit of prior planning and a great deal of ease.

Plane Attire

Wear a comfortable suit, preferably a skirt with an elastic waistband in a fabric that will keep its shape such as wool serge, a poly and linen viscose, or a rayon blend. The latter doesn't keep its shape so much as it comes in styles that don't cry out for pressed pleats. Once on the plane, fold the suit jacket into an overhead rack to keep it from wrinkling.

If pants are acceptable in your company, and you prefer them to a skirt, then by all means wear a beautiful imported rayon or tropical-weight wool pants suit on the aircraft.

Don't wear your most dressy silk blouse for travel, as they can't tolerate an ounce of perspiration. Wear a handsome blend that withstands wrinkling and which can, if absolutely necessary, even be rinsed out in a hotel sink on arrival.

Sporting a special scarf? Fold it into your carryon or into a tote after boarding. Put it on again as you make your final descent, then slip on the suit jacket.

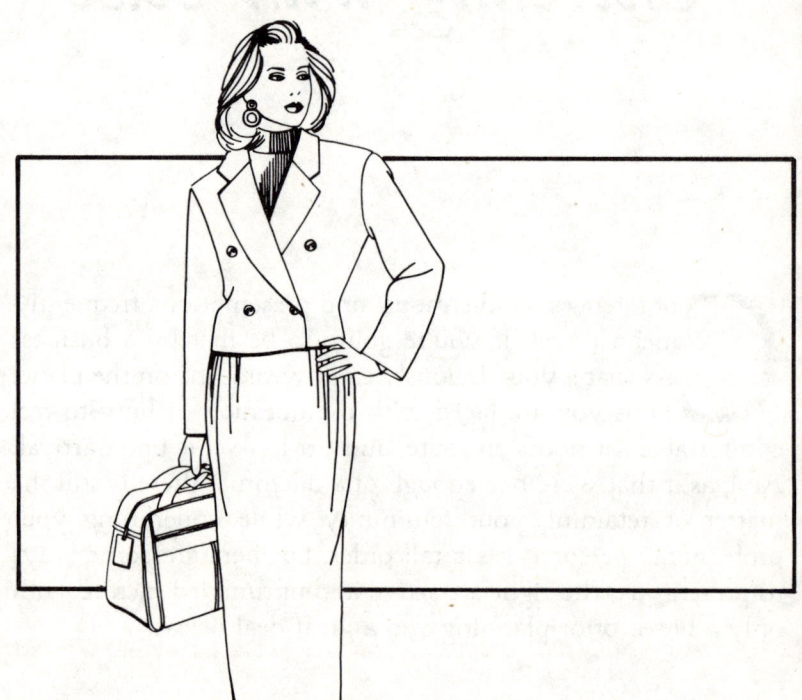

Noncrushables

Choose fabrics when traveling and packing that won't wrinkle easily. No matter how that linen suit tempts you (unless you want to have it pressed all over again at the hotel) stay away. Take silky, luxurious polyblend shirts. Cotton or synthetic knits, and tissue-weight wool gabardine also travel uncrushably. You may need to have the hotel laundry service touch up some items lightly with an iron, but then again the creases may just uncrease when hung nearby as you shower.

Traveling Light

Pack around two basic neutral colors: black and white, beige and brown, gray and blue, or purple and black, so that every basic garment you bring works with everything else. Then pick out lightweight, colorful accessories.

For a week's trip bring:

- two jackets (one of them a blazer)
- two skirts
- a pair of pants
- four blouses
- a camisole
- a dressy sweater (unless you're heading into hot weather)
- a dressy blouse
- five pair of pantyhose
- one pair of medium-heeled shoes
- a higher-heeled pair

"I put plastic over the things I'm taking, blouse, suit, then put them into a garment bag and that keeps them from wrinkling. Or in the suitcase, I fold them with the plastic bag still on them, and hangers intact. Or I wrap clothes in tissue paper, but that's harder to come by."

Director of Purchasing

If you think you'll need it, include a trench coat. Include necklaces, pins, scarves, and perhaps a hair ornament.

Keep a toiletries bag of miniatures ready in a carry-on bag so that you don't have to concern yourself with these details every time you make a business trip. Be sure to include shower sandals. From time to time, update the contents to make sure you still have a shower cap, toothpaste, lipstick, and deodorant.

Pack in layers. Put heavy things on the bottom with shoes first in plastic bags. Fit underwear around them. Pack shirts flat in their plastic dry cleaners' bags. Hang skirts, jackets, and dresses in a garment bag which you can stow in a forward compartment on the airplane.

For lightweight touches that provide a change in your basic outfits, bring a camisole to add flair to a suit for dinner meetings, a chiffon scarf to turn a daytime look into nighttime chic, and shoe clips to glamorize basic pumps for evening wear.

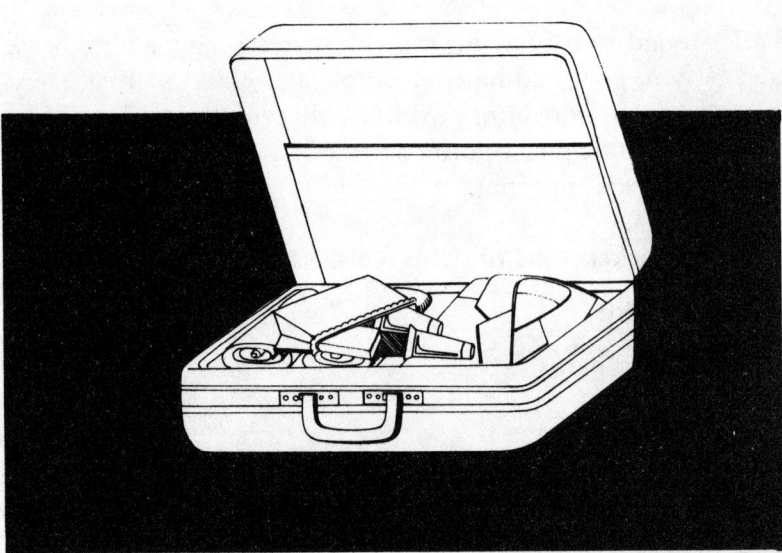

You do want to take a tiny travel alarm clock unless your watch has an alarm. Even though you can get a wake-up call from the desk, this is not foolproof. It also doesn't tell you the time on a regular basis.

Carrying On

To safeguard against luggage going astray, it is a good idea to carry certain items with you. Important business papers, a tape recorder for dictating, eyeglasses, pens, sunglasses, or spare contact lenses and lens kit should not be checked. A large scarf or stole is good to have available on the plane in case the air-conditioning system is in high gear.

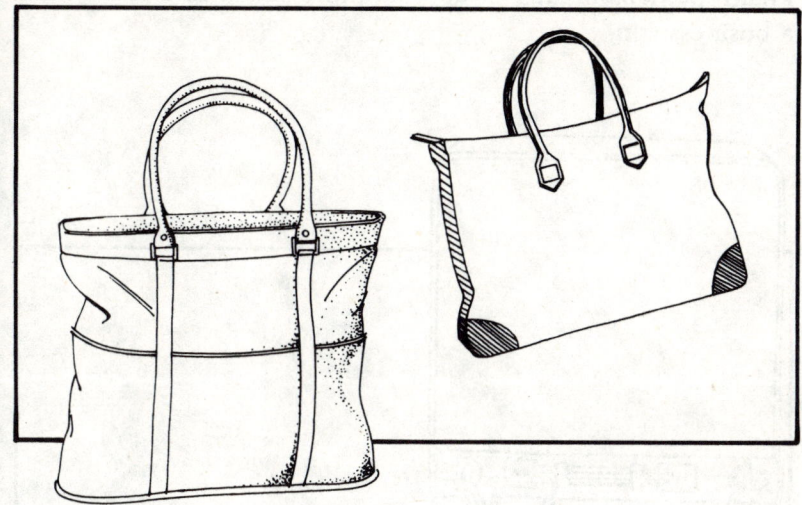

"I travel with a lot of dresses, so when I get to my hotel, I hang them in the shower right away. Usually I also have to call down for an iron, though, to touch them up."

Fashion Representative

If possible it's wise to include in your carryon anything you think you might need for one full day in case your luggage goes on to Seattle while you disembark in Houston.

Bags

Above all, don't travel with dowdy-looking bags. Some nylon and woven nylon Pullman-style luggage comes with a frame which protects clothing in transit far better than the unstructured bags. Shaped leather bags are expensive but they look great and they carry clothes and other items more safely than unstructured nylon. They are, however, going to get marred and scarred by handling. Nylon and woven nylon (which is reportedly tougher) bags come in a wide range of colors and patterns. They are lightweight, resilient, and do not show wear and tear easily. Stripes are a good choice—floral is possibly a little too feminine, although it might be just fine if you're in the fashion field or some other creative spot.

Good colors for the businesswoman's luggage are teal, black, and camel. Red or plum work very well in clothing, but somehow as luggage they seem more at home in the Caribbean. Another color which does not translate well into luggage is khaki, perhaps because it appears more suited to a safari than a business trip.

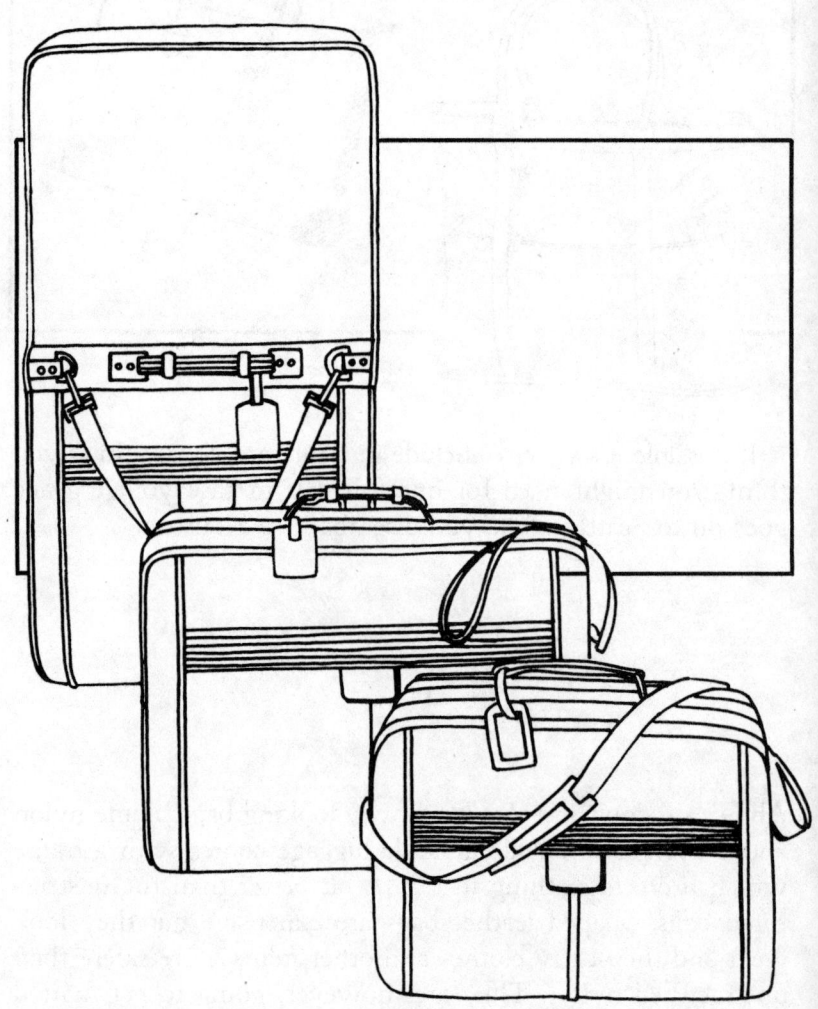

Traveling Ease

For a one-week trip, take a tote of business papers or a carryon, a garment bag, and a small Pullman. For a two-day trip, a Pullman and a tote should handle everything sufficiently. A garment bag will keep dresses and suits relatively neat and can be checked or carried on board. A tote can serve as a carryon, as a purse, and briefcase. While a briefcase looks impressively handsome, many women, especially when traveling, opt for tote bags because they offer room for a spare pair of shoes, perhaps slip-on rain totes, and a makeup purse in addition to business papers. Totes are just as attractive as briefcases, they're not as mannish, and they're great for travel.

"Nylon bags are light; however, some of them are expensive, and also it's no fun to arrive with crumpled clothing. I prefer a leather bag with boxy construction."

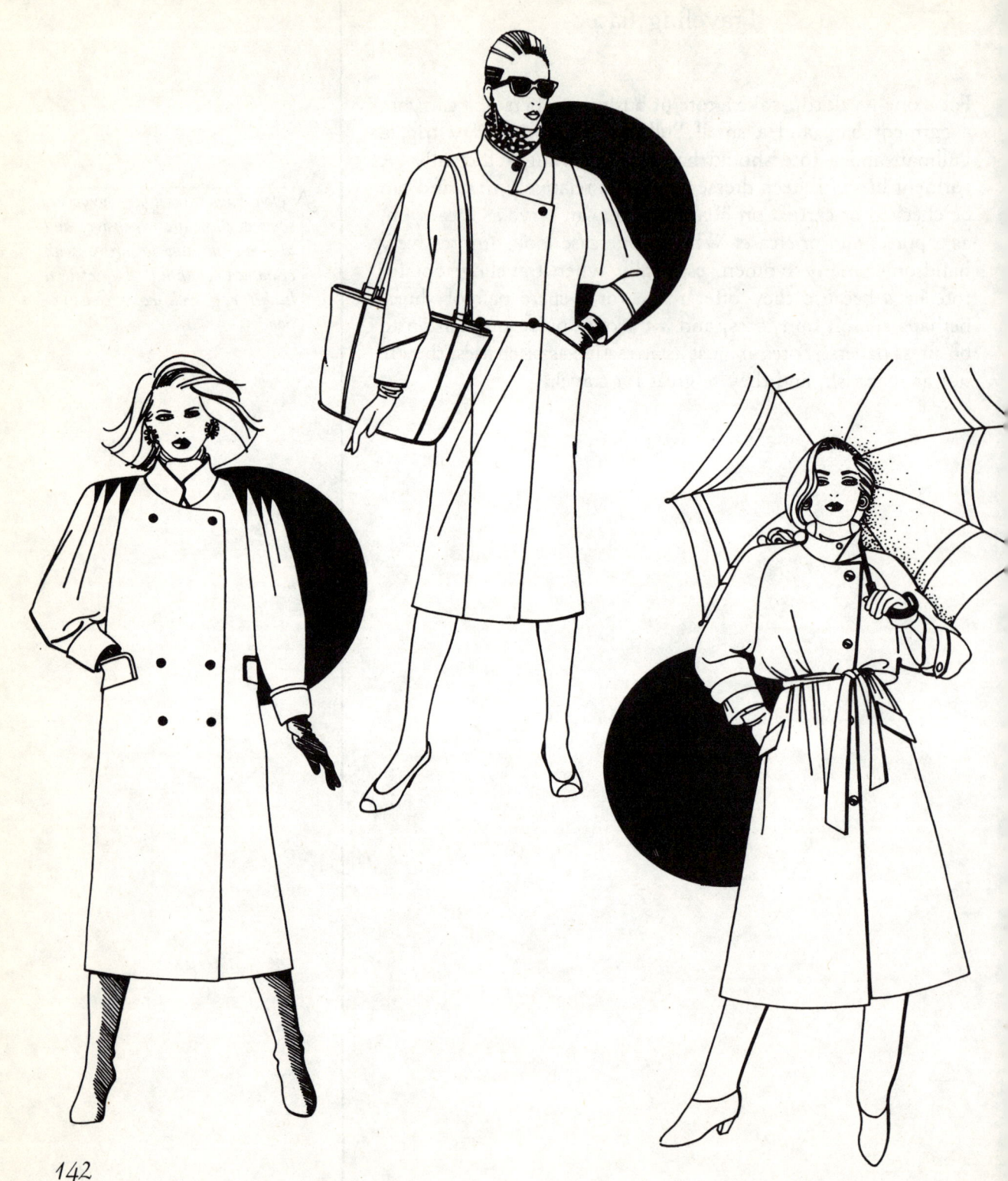

CHAPTER 11

Foul Weather Gear

There's nothing like looking bedraggled to ruin your chances at winning over a client or interviewer. However, neither rain, sleet, or snow is any match for a little advanced planning. There are plenty of great-looking and versatile possibilities out there to help you keep looking unruffled no matter the weather. And to make matters even "sunnier," most such garments can also be worn in beautiful weather. The result? No wasted money, and plenty of lovely looks for any day of the year.

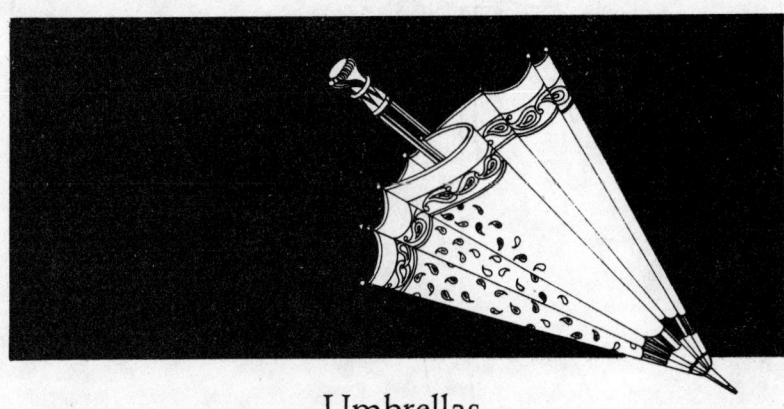

Umbrellas

The umbrella you choose should be one that says "class." How about a splendidly large Italian paisley to go with those checks and plaid outfits, and one with a beautifully carved malacca handle.

Rain Gear

Invest in a fine raincoat, one that is cut generously enough to go over a suit, and is long enough to cover a mid-calf skirt so that you don't have a skirt layering out from the bottom. Do look for one that is water-repellent, not merely water-resistant, since it is supposed to be a raincoat after all.

A basically beige raincoat with a light floral lining, standup collar, lightly lined, can make you feel good on rainy days. It

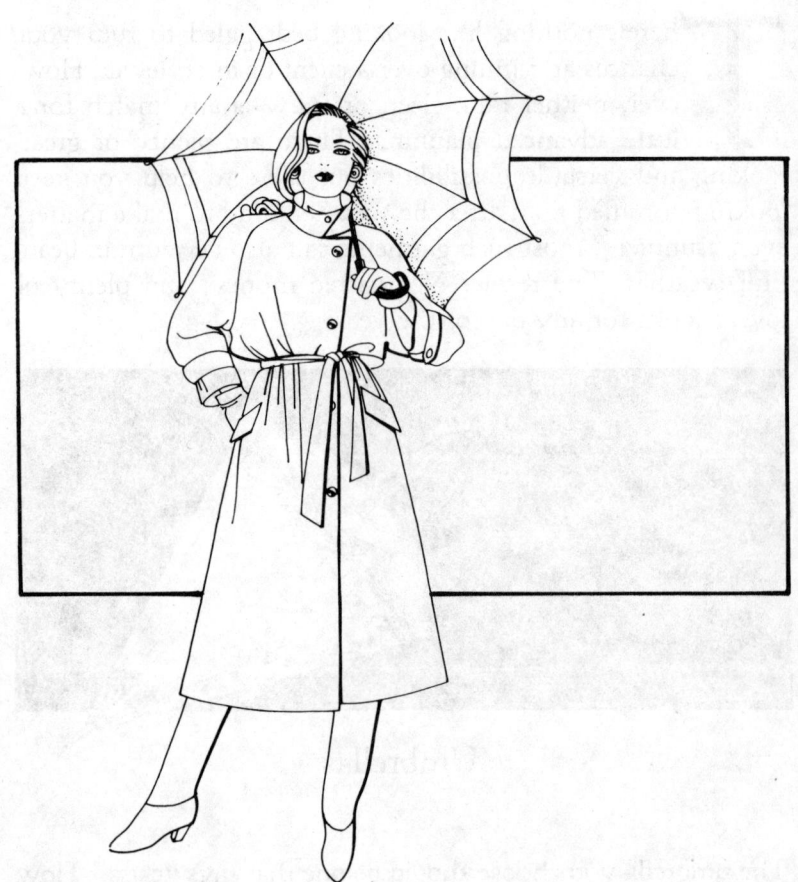

is neutral enough to be professionally acceptable, but feminine enough to suit your new approach to fashion. It's best to wear no rain hat with this one; just carry an equally elegant umbrella.

- Polyurethane laminated over either cotton or polyester makes for one of those eerily luminescent raincoats that looks as though it should glow in the dark (but doesn't). It looks as now as a laser and offers a chic alternative to the khaki matte look of a trench coat.

- Rubberized cotton is waterproof and can also look chic, believe it or not, *if* it's made into a riding-style cropped A-line coat. Wear it with natural chamois gloves.

- Raincoats can be as intriguing as they are practically serious. A cotton water-repellent coat with a zip-out lining is probably the most versatile of all outergear, and goes anywhere that business takes you. To avoid that severe mannish cast, add a vivid striped, paisley, or floral fringed scarf with it.

- Brave rain or shine in a water-repellent black satin coat. It can be dressed up for night or looks satisfactorily commanding for daytime wear.

Lighten up the seriousness of coats for all weather with a range of colorful scarves: plaid, paisley, hairline stripes, pindots, double stripe, heraldic or geometric print, floral, vine pattern, horsey pattern, dog motif. The choices in scarves are wide and will help lend you that personalized career look.

Winter Coats

Winter coats present a major investment even in wools with no fur trim. Some of the best coat styles include trench, reefer, chesterfield, and wrap because they're classic and never seem to go out of style, plus they provide room for you to wear a suit underneath. A perfectly tailored camel overcoat goes every-

"I wear a waterproof shiny black fabric fashionable coat and high waterproof boots in the rain; actually, I wear that outfit in snow more than rain."
Personnel Manager

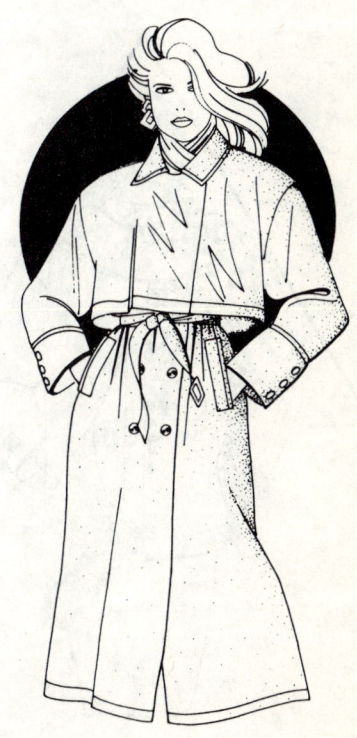

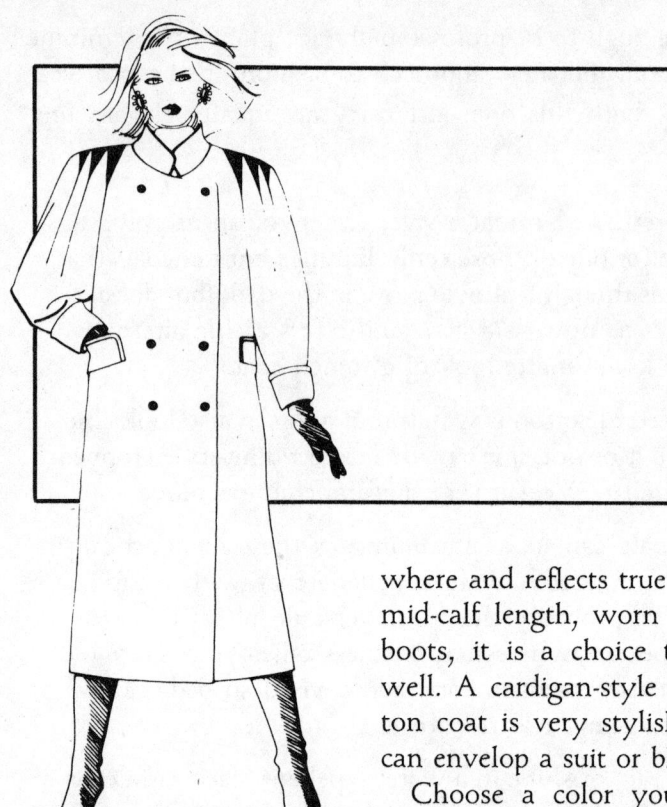

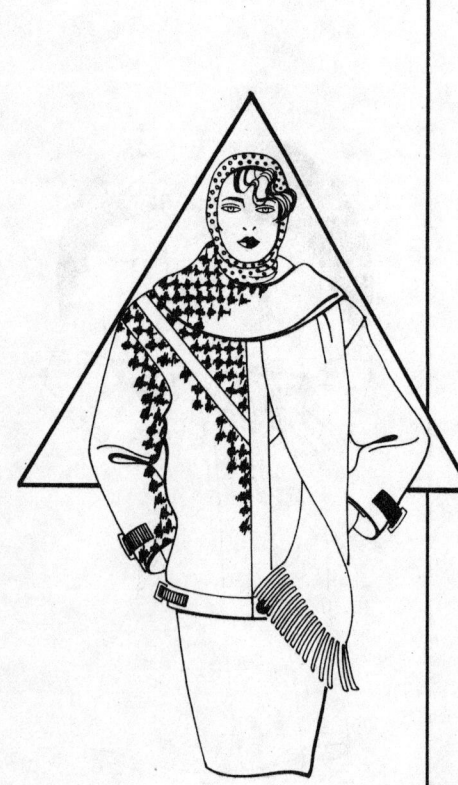

where and reflects true class. In a mid-calf length, worn with high boots, it is a choice that wears well. A cardigan-style single button coat is very stylish and also can envelop a suit or blazer.

Choose a color you can live with for many seasons and simple lines that will not quickly lose style. Loden green is successful in a double-breasted English wool overcoat. Warm *and* very stylish. Pigskin gloves lined in cashmere set off this type of coat. Fuchsia as a color undoubtedly won't remain in style longer than a few seasons.

Some otherwise quite plain coats have small details which set them off, such as leather gussets or wide puffed sleeves. You might not mind investing in a deep dark color if you can find a silhouette that pleases.

Plums, bright blues, and pinks are now a real treat in formerly dark only winter coats. Before buying, ask yourself: Will I be happy with plum two years from now? You may be. Then again, that vivid a hue could grow quickly tiresome.

A houndstooth jacket with a wide fringed self stole and jersey hood is one way to skirt the long-length coat and still look terrific.

Length

You will want your coats longer than your skirts; that means to below the knee or even mid-calf, which is the most practical length of all. For a short, short coat, the broad-shaped cocoon style comes to mid-knee to accommodate the shorter hemline look. In some shops they are labeled "jackets." You'll recognize them because they look almost fingertip length, an alternative to the mid-calf hemline. The problem with this shorter length is that it cannot be worn with any garment longer than it is, plus when it goes out of style, there is no way to adjust the hemline.

- If you already have your basic heavy coat and want something special, try a chocolate-colored quilted leather for a new look. It would look exquisite with a paisley print scarf with long delicate fringes.

- Don't forget capes as another alternative. They easily go over suits, especially shoulder capes, and look and feel dramatic, although they are not as warm as a button-up coat.

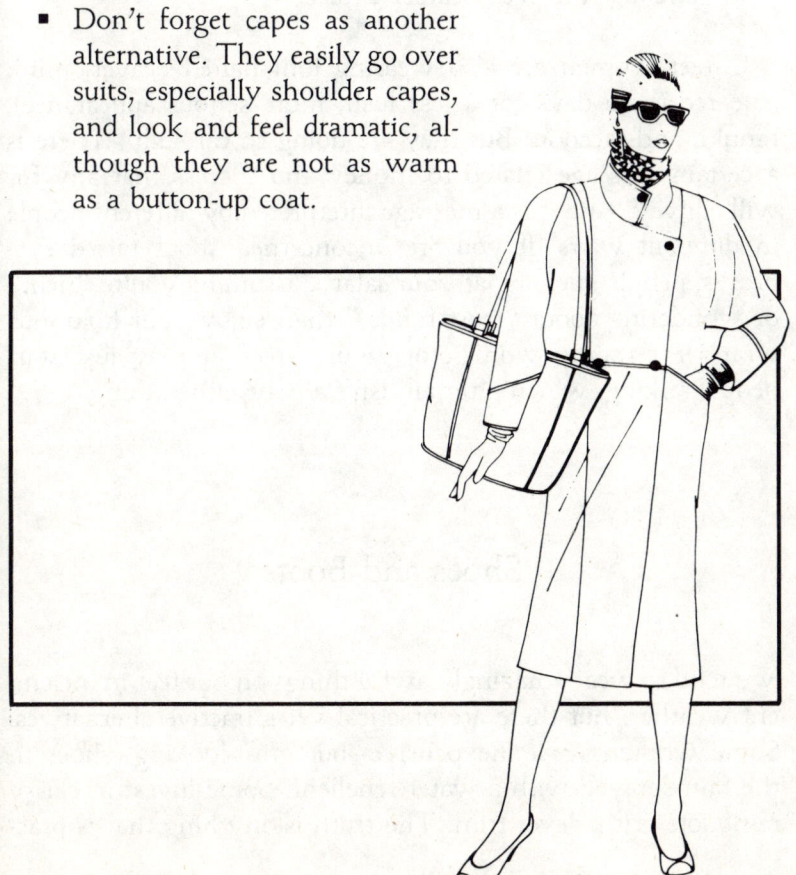

- A chic compromise between sheer elegance and practicality—a silk gabardine coat. The texture alone is worth the price.

- If the coat you like has pedestrian buttons, try to picture it with large, expensive ones which could make all the difference, but would mean only about another ten-dollar investment to you.

- This is where leather comes into play, too, in a full-length simple style with a high neck, matching gloves—nothing could be more understated and yet impressive.

- Should you go fur-trimmed in a daytime work coat? There is no reason not to, if you like the coat and it fits your career. The variety of fur-trimmed coats ranges from modestly simple to very dressy. Modestly simple in a classic style large enough to accommodate a suit is generally the better career choice.

Career women are also wearing long-haired beaver, mink (sheared these days for a less lush, more serious appearance), tanuki, and raccoon. But they are doing so carefully. There is a certain message related to money and success that any fur will convey. And it is a message interpreted by different people in different ways. If you are unconcerned about raised eyebrows, people guessing at your salary, assuming you're "rich," or wondering about "trust funds," than enjoy your luxurious wrap. It certainly won't stop your career. It may just start people talking, which after all, isn't always a bad thing.

Shoes and Boots

We tend to wear amazingly awful things on our feet in inclement weather. But there are practical yet attractive alternatives. Some women wear inexpensive—but great-looking—shoes in the rain sprayed with a water repellent. Some invest in classy rainboots with clever trim. The truth is anything that is practical yet neat is quite acceptable in the business world. See-through plastic slip-ons that go over shoes do protect expensive leather from being totally destroyed in an unforecast shower. They can be carried in a tote bag, too, and slipped on and off unobtrusively.

Then there is snow. High leather boots look fantastic, especially with a mid-calf coat. But they can't take much snow, even with so-called water-proofing treatment. That leaves us with a choice of not quite so chic-looking but more practical footwear. Choices are improving as new fabrics come onto the market, however, and in a small heel, some truly waterproof, matte-finish boots are available. They come lined so they are also warmer than totally rubber boots which do not look as dressy.

Hats

Anything that covers the head to some degree is going to help keep you warm in winter. Fur earmuffs are one way to go. They don't mess the hair and they do keep the ears warm. Pretty, colorful classic berets look good, and keep the top of the head warm, but don't do much for the ears. Knit hats look a little too casual, although a heavy crocheted, oversized beret with a pretty clip or pin can look lovely at the same time as it is practical. Men's-style hats in felt or wool look dressy as well as professional.

Dos and Don'ts

Do

Tie a bright neck scarf into a bow to dress up the collar of a raincoat.

Wear fur or wool headbands over ears. These will not flatten or electrify the hair, and they look very flapper-ish and chic.

Drape a long, wool challis scarf around the shoulders of your coat.

Add color with knit mufflers, long, thick, and vivid.

Go for fleece-lined rubber boots to cover cold rainy days and snow.

Choose a high leather boot for cold days.

Try long-line gloves in funky colors.

Wear a silk or cotton camisole beneath blouses to maintain warmth and to absorb perspiration.

Don't

Think people are not going to notice what you wear on bad-weather days.

Choose raincoats that are merely water-resistant, unless you plan to wear them only in dry weather.

Wear good leather boots in slush and snow. They will stain, among other things.

Overdress. Layer so that you can remove items in order to cool off quickly when you enter a building or a commuter train.

Combine an angora scarf with a black coat. You will never remove all of the lint.

Let a skirt show below your coat. Buy a coat shorter than the longest hemline in your wardrobe.

Buy a snug-fitting coat that doesn't allow room for a jacket.

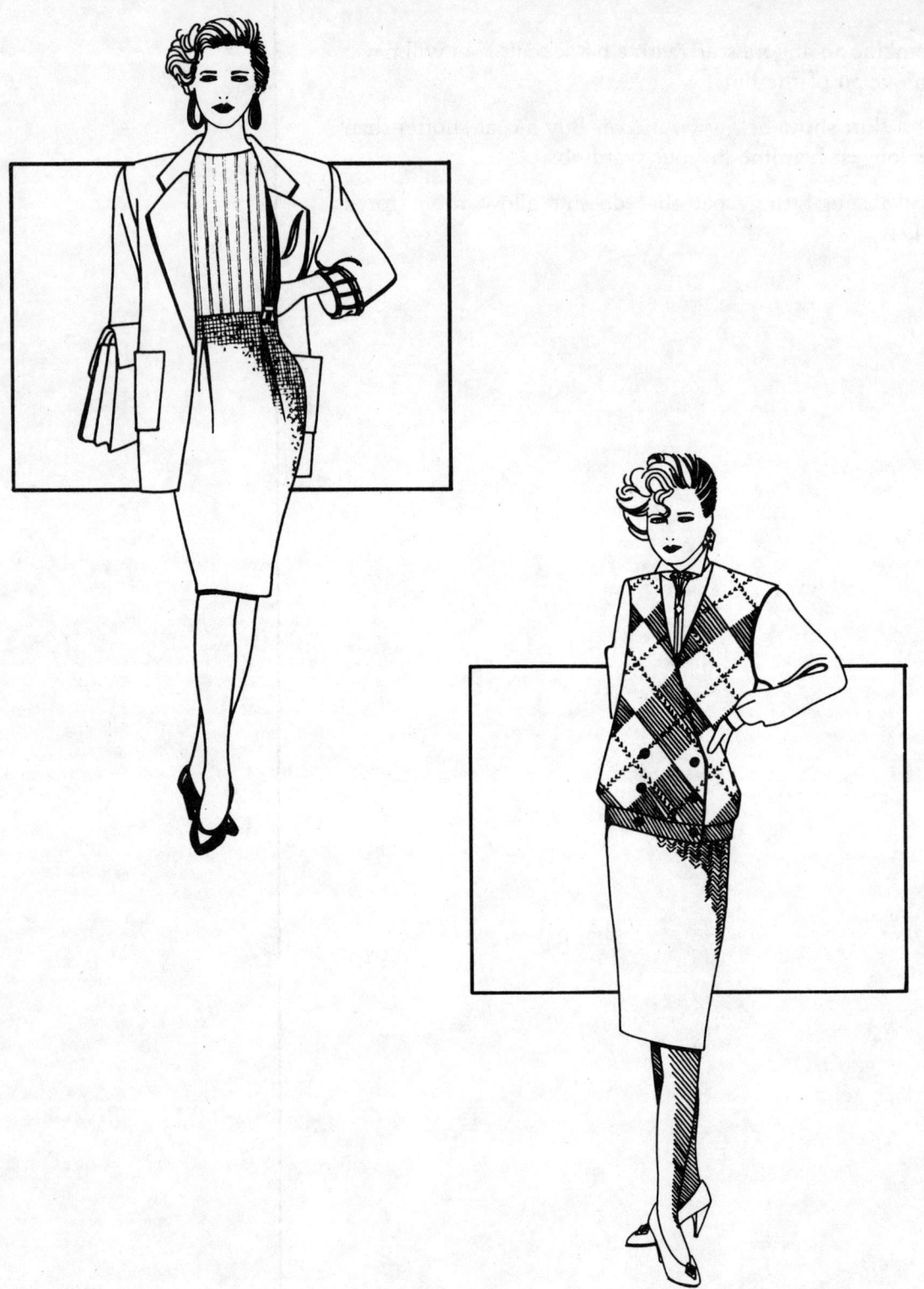

CHAPTER

12

Outfits You Never Dreamed You Could Wear

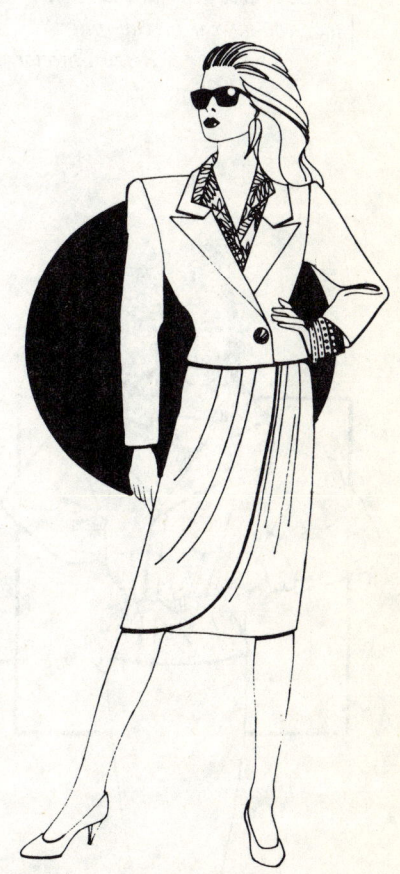

Here are some unusual items that you would never dream you could wear on the job, but when teamed creatively with a selection of more standard fare, they make for a unique and individualistic fashion statement that is at once savvy *and* chic.

HAWAIIAN SHIRT: Worn with a sarong-style jersey skirt with a three-chain belt and a short-cropped jacket, this can be a successful business/fashion look. Perfect for advertising sales.

ARGYLE SOCKS: If they are silky, and paired with a herringbone or gray wool suit with pumps, you can look gorgeous for banking or accounting.

BOMBER LEATHER JACKET: Over a slim skirt, silk skirt, one-tone hose and pumps, and gold chains, this would work well in teaching, advertising (perfect), or fashion.

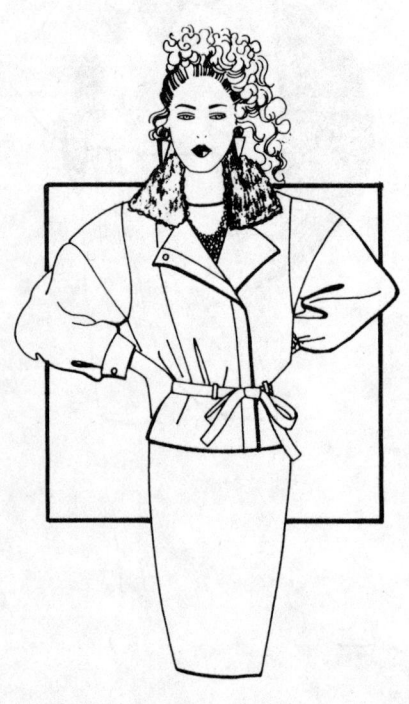

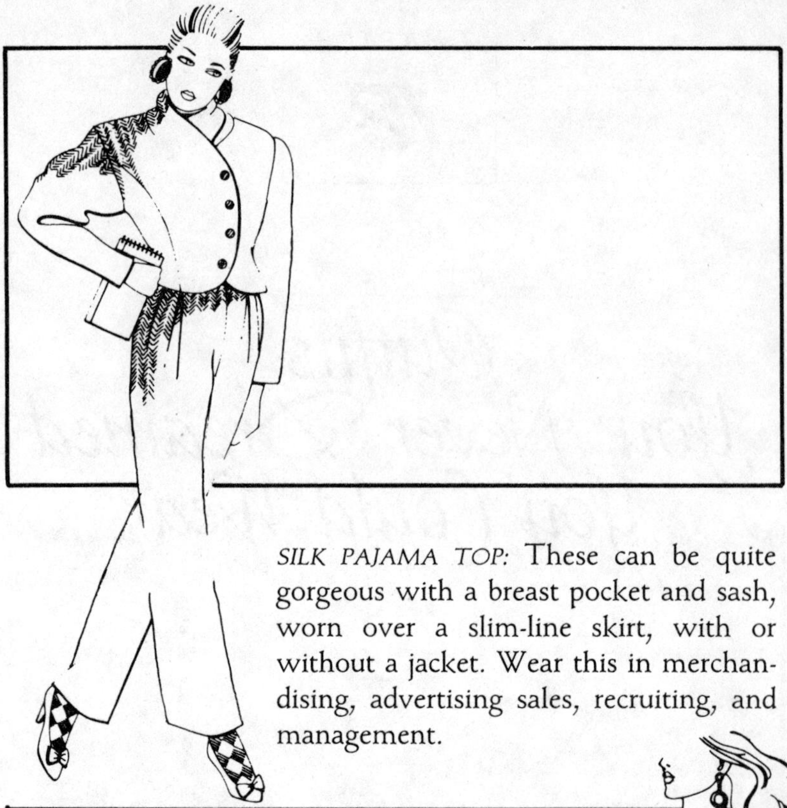

SILK PAJAMA TOP: These can be quite gorgeous with a breast pocket and sash, worn over a slim-line skirt, with or without a jacket. Wear this in merchandising, advertising sales, recruiting, and management.

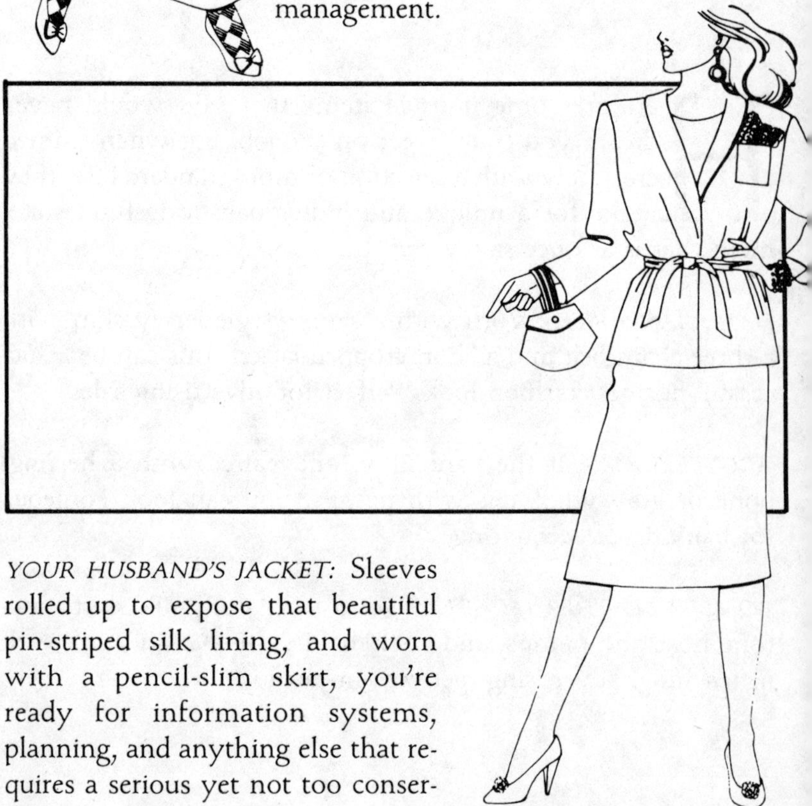

YOUR HUSBAND'S JACKET: Sleeves rolled up to expose that beautiful pin-striped silk lining, and worn with a pencil-slim skirt, you're ready for information systems, planning, and anything else that requires a serious yet not too conservative look with style.

154

HIS SWEATER VEST: This can be worn under a suit or to make up a mismatched-suit effect (sans jacket). Big, blousy, preferably cashmere, this outfit can be worn in accounting, banking, law, budgeting, or teaching. It is an attractive maternity look as well.

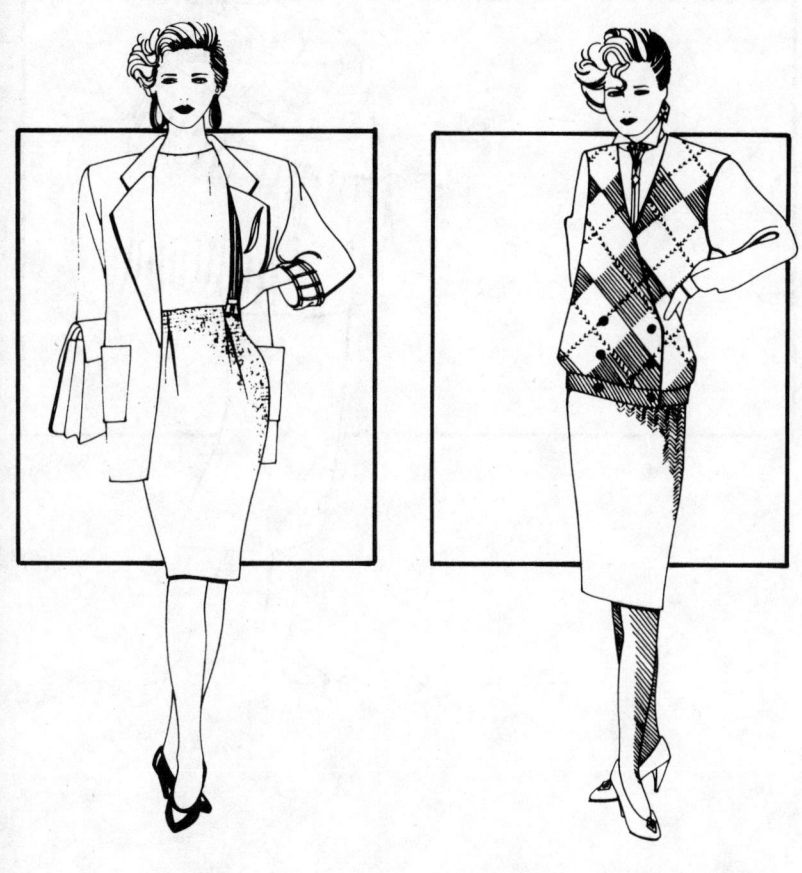

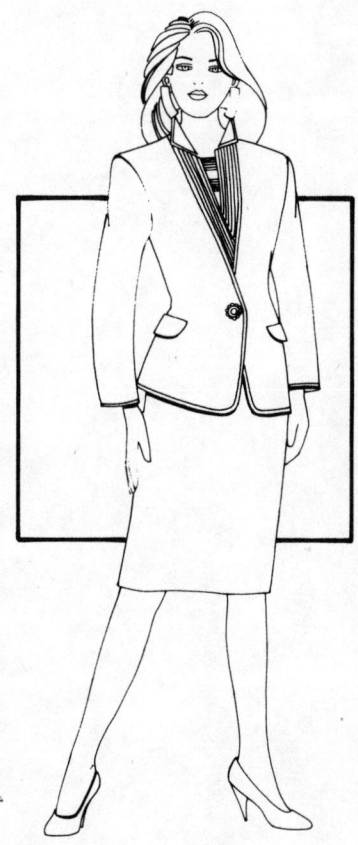

STRIPED LEOTARD UNDER A WHITE SHIRT: For a touch of color—getting away from the typical scarf—wear a vivid workout leotard under a crisp, tuxedo-style white shirt with a mismatched or matched suit. This is great for teaching, design, or even accounting.

155

BLANKET: For a cool-weather stole, a thick, wooly stadium-size blanket with fringe can be the perfect accompaniment to a subdued, chic suit. This would work for all professions, from the most conservative to the creative.